THE SHAAR PRESS

THE JUDAICA IMPRINT
FOR THOUGHTFUL PEOPLE

U P W

THE SHAAR PRESS

SHAMI REINMAN

ARDS

The story of my struggle with Parkinsonism

First edition – First impression / March 2014

Published by **SHAAR PRESS**
Distributed by MESORAH PUBLICATIONS, LTD.
4401 Second Avenue / Brooklyn, N.Y 11232 / (718) 921-9000

Distributed in Israel by SIFRIATI / A. GITLER
Moshav Magshimim / Israel

Distributed in Europe by LEHMANNS
Unit E, Viking Business Park, Rolling Mill Road / Jarrow, Tyne and Wear, NE32 3DP/ England

Distributed in Australia and New Zealand by GOLDS WORLD OF JUDAICA
3-13 William Street / Balaclava, Melbourne 3183 / Victoria Australia

Distributed in South Africa by KOLLEL BOOKSHOP
Northfield Centre / 17 Northfield Avenue / Glenhazel 2192, Johannesburg, South Africa

ISBN 10: 1-4226-1479-4 / ISBN 13: 978-1-4226-1479-2

Printed in the United States of America
Custom bound by Sefercraft, Inc. / 4401 Second Avenue / Brooklyn N.Y. 11232

Table of Contents

Springtime in Manhattan

On a beautiful April day in 2006, we were driving along the upper level of the George Washington Bridge. Yossel, my husband, was at the wheel, and I was gazing through the window. Below us, the Hudson River sparkled in the sun. Yossel pointed to the tall buildings in the distance, on the eastern shore of the river. Those buildings, he said, were Columbia Presbyterian Hospital. Never having seen them, I looked at them now with a mixture of dread and hope.

We were both apprehensive and didn't talk much as we crossed the river. My thigh and the big toe on my right foot were throbbing with pain. I squirmed in my seat, trying to find a more comfortable position, but there was none. No matter how I sat, the pain did not let up. I'd been struggling with these symptoms for two years. I'd seen a general practitioner, a sports orthopedist, a cardiologist, a podiatrist, a few chiropractors, and a holistic healer, and none of them had done much to help. Now we were coming to Columbia Presbyterian. Would we find the answer here? Would this agony finally come to an end?

We exited the bridge and turned into Fort Washington Avenue, with the hospital up ahead. The sun was shining. The air was soft and warm. I was out with my husband, and we always enjoy our time together. We were planning to go to lunch in Teaneck afterward, hopefully to celebrate the discovery of the solution to my problems. My husband was optimistic, as he usually is. Me? I'm the more realistic one.

Our appointment was in the Milstein Pavilion. The main entrance is on Fort Washington Avenue. A curved driveway cuts into the building under the first floor. The driveway was jammed with cars and vans and ambulances. Pulling over on the left side, Yossel opened the trunk and took out the MRIs and X-rays from the previous two years; it was quite a package. He gave the keys to an attendant, and we turned back onto the avenue.

It was close to lunchtime, and there were many people rushing about. Most of them were easily identifiable as doctors, nurses, orderlies or other hospital personnel. The rest were probably patients, like me. On the corner across the street was a kiosk where one could purchase newspapers, magazines and bottled water. A little beyond, were two pushcarts laden with fresh fruits and vegetables.

We turned the corner toward the river. A cement ramp, at least fifty feet long, ran alongside the building. There were steps, but we didn't see anyone use them. Most were taking the ramp, as it was the shortest distance between the avenue and the door. We did the same.

A security guard sat at a desk inside the small lobby, under a sign that said Department of Neurology. Our appointment was with Dr. David Adams, and the guard directed us to the sixth floor. We signed in and sat down. I looked around at the other people waiting, worried about meeting someone I knew. It would have been so embarrassing. Fortunately, I didn't see anyone who looked Orthodox.

I turned to my husband. "What do you think he's going to say,

Yossel?" His name is Yaakov Yosef. About fifteen years ago, he decided that he prefers being called by his full name, though close family still call him Yossel. "Do you think he'll say it's the Lipitor?" I took that medication to lower my cholesterol.

"I can't even begin to guess what he's going to say. I can't even think about it." That's him. He doesn't want to think about anything negative unless he has no choice. But I'm always thinking of the worst. Yossel used to travel to New York once a week and if the weather was bad, I would think what if there was an accident and he was killed, Heaven forbid. What would I do? How would I cope? It's not that I'm not afraid to think of bad things; it's that I can't help it. My mind works that way.

So what was I thinking now? Well, what wasn't I thinking? To be realistic, I am generally a positive person, and I was really hoping that everything would work out fine.

Asked to describe my personality, I'd have said that I've basically been a happy-go-lucky, fun-loving person all my life. I didn't do that well scholastically, but I loved the school spirit, the friendships, the songs, the sheer fun of it all. And that is why I really loved summer camp. It had all the fun of school and none of the work. I was always ready for adventure.

My first camp experience was in Camp Naarah, in the Catskill Mountains. My older sister was a regular camper there, and my family was spending the summer nearby. Wanting to keep me busy, my mother pleaded with Mrs. Stubenhaus, the camp's director, to accept me as a day camper.

I was only five-and-a-half years old at the time, while the girls in the bunk were six. After a few days, I asked my mother to let me sleep in the camp like everyone else. My mother was doubtful, but I begged and begged.

"Let her try it," Mrs. Stubenhaus told my mother. "Don't worry. She'll come running home after one night."

She was wrong. I became the youngest camper and loved every minute of it. At home, my sister and I had often staged performances in front of the mirror, or for our immediate family; in camp, we would stand on two big chairs and sing for the whole camp on Friday nights. We were quite a hit. I was hav-

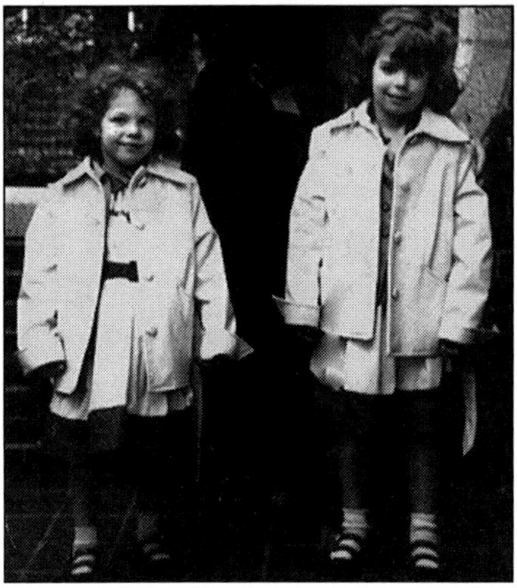

Shami and her sister as little girls

ing the time of my life. Every night, I fell into my bunk exhausted and slept like a baby.

School was another story. I was not, as I've said, the greatest student. I've always felt that I started school too early. I was the youngest in my class. It's all right to embark on summer camp when you're barely out of diapers, but school is different. School is serious, which I never was. I never did take myself too seriously, and through my struggles with my disease, this became my biggest strength.

But I still craved attention, so I became a bit of a troublemaker, in a nice way, of course. There was the time, in the fourth

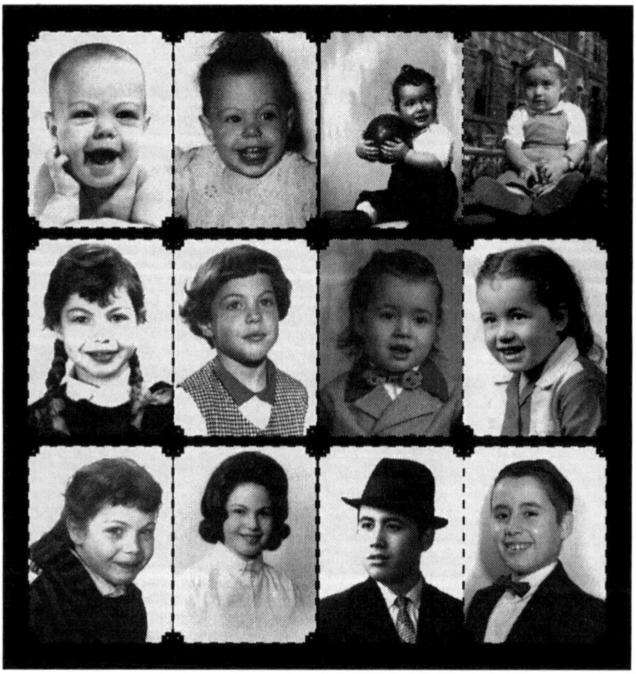

Collage of photos of the author and her husband as they were growing up. Collage prepared by the author.

grade, when I bent a paper clip and shaped it over my teeth so that it looked like a bite plate. My teacher, seeing how uncomfortable I was in my "new braces," gave me aspirin and cold compresses. Little did she know that it was the edges of the paperclip poking into my cheeks that were causing the discomfort.

Once, in the eighth grade, I was coming out of the bathroom when I saw the principal and the teacher outside our classroom door.

"Shami Rubin, you'd better unlock this door!" they shouted.

I came over and stood behind them. I was in tears.

"Is that what you think of me?" I asked. "I would never lock a teacher out of a classroom! I might crack jokes or do silly things, but I would never do such a thing." I had some mischief in me, but I was never disrespectful.

By the time I reached high school, I was known as the class wit, always cracking one-liners and getting thrown out of class for my efforts. The administration did not make fine distinctions; a troublemaker was a troublemaker, period.

It wasn't until eleventh grade that I finally realized that school was interesting. By then, I had to study hard just to pass.

So it was not surprising that I had a bad case of cold feet when my husband and I became engaged. All the Reinmans are so brilliant. How would I fit in?

Luckily, I had my sense of humor. The one-liners that would repeatedly get me in trouble in class saved me on the night I met his family. I told jokes. I was funny. Everyone liked me. It was a miracle.

I once told Yossel that I felt bad about not knowing algebra or geometry, but he didn't think it was such a big deal. To make me happy, he taught them to me over lunch in two weeks.

After we were married, I was a teacher and a mother, and spent many summers as a lifeguard and nurse in the summer camps I loved. Always, fun was my middle name. I enjoyed playing practical jokes and being the life of the party. But even more I loved bringing out the best in people. That side of me came out strongly in raising a family and as a teacher.

I had a full life, a husband I admired, bright and creative chil-

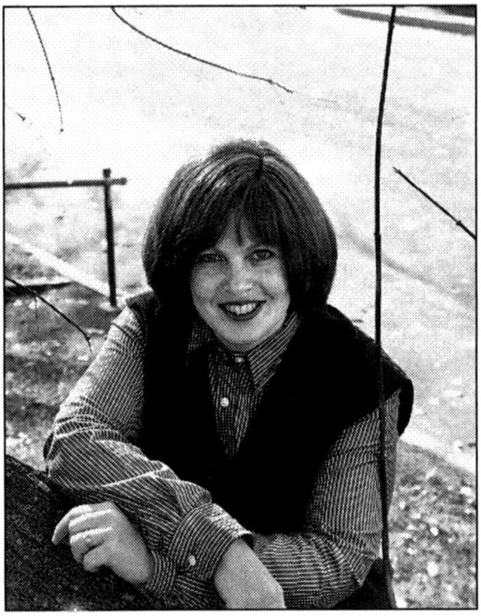

The author as a teacher

dren and wonderful grandchildren, and I loved my work. I taught First Aid and Computers; I wrote safety pamphlets and computer workbooks. I bonded with my students in Bais Kaila and Ilan and used my computer savvy to help them be confident and creative. Whatever they were into, I was into. Those were my healthy years .

After our kids were grown, we moved to a different neighborhood in the same town, Lakewood, New Jersey. Our new house had a large swimming pool in the backyard, where I swam laps every chance I got. Most of our neighbors were quite a bit younger, and they were curious about the new people moving in .

One of them asked a friend of mine, "Who is this grandmother moving to our block?"

"Grandmother?" my friend replied. "Just try and keep up with her."

As a grandmother, I was in my element. I loved every project or hobby that my grandchildren were engaged in. They knew that nothing was too childish or boring for me. My eyes would light up with the same brightness that theirs did. I would read through instructions, figure out how to download music, do puzzles and play board games .

My oldest grandson, Shmuel, was very inquisitive. I lovingly would sit with him at the computer for hours, showing him different graphics programs to keep him entertained. At four years old, he called and asked, "Bobby, can I come play CorelDraw with you?" We created our very own storybook. The kids are my best friends, and they know it. I am one of them, and we love life together.

Now, things were changing. The problem was slowly evolving, and the active Shami was gone. The fullness of my life was now defined by aches, pains and anxiety.

It began with the pain in my toes. I couldn't straighten them, and when a shoe pressed against the top of my foot, twinges would shoot from the toe right up to my ankle. At night, if I hit my toes against the blanket the pain would be strong enough to wake me. I needed to find out what was wrong with me, and so began my journey into the medical maze of my illness.

I went to see Dr. Brian Halpern, a sports orthopedist who had been recommended by a neighbor. He took x-rays to see if any toes were fractured. The pictures showed nothing. Two weeks later, in mid-June, 2004, in desperation, I visited a local podiatrist. He injected cortisone directly into my toes. I saw stars and was conscious of a spongy feeling in my toes — but the pain was gone.

Unfortunately, the relief was only temporary.

The symptoms persisted. And worsened.

By August, my back beneath the shoulder blades began hurting. I felt that my posture was distorted. It was as if my body was being pushed forward, forcing me to walk like a hunchback. I found myself watching the ground instead of seeing the leaves on the trees.

Taking a walk one morning, my heart seemed to be skipping beats. Terrified, I called my primary physician, who sent me to Dr. Bacharach, a cardiologist. I underwent a stress test and had dye injected into my veins so that my heart function could be monitored. All seemed fine.

At that time, the lease was up on our car, and it took quite a while to find a car that suited me in my new condition. Most cars are not built for short people. I generally find the driver's seat too long in front and tilted downward at the back. But this was not the ordinary discomfort of driving in a car intended for a taller person. On the thirty-minute drive to school each day, I would have to massage my thigh as I drove, to try and loosen up the muscle. I would adjust my seat in different ways, in an effort to ease the spasms. On one occasion, my leg muscles became so tight that I had to stop at the side of the road and rest because I was afraid I wouldn't be able to hit the brake pedal when necessary.

I tried using my left foot on the brake to give my right thigh a rest, but this wasn't practical. The more I tried to relax, the more tense my thigh became. It was hard for me to change positions in the car. If I slipped into the driver's seat and needed to smooth down my skirt, I found that I couldn't lift myself to do so. Most of the time, I was too dizzy to drive.

One morning, I was putting on my seatbelt when I began feeling more out of sorts than usual. I stopped at a gas station to fill up, but had difficulty taking my wallet out of my pocketbook. The attendant waited patiently for what seemed like half an hour as I emptied my entire contents of my bag, until I finally located my wallet and handed him the credit card.

After that, I tried getting rides to school. This was impractical, as I had various responsibilities at school that often kept me after hours. On the days I wasn't teaching, I tried resting in bed. This helped somewhat, but left me feeling impatient and frustrated. I'm not the resting type.

As a teacher, my voice was very important to me. To my dismay, that was the next thing to go. As my vocal cords began to lose their strength, it became harder and harder to project my voice. I invested two hundred dollars in a microphone system for the computer lab. The speakers were in the back of the room, where two students sat. The sound was tinny and very annoying for them.

I had a meeting with my principal one afternoon. My difficulty speaking clearly was becoming a real issue. I was so nervous that I wouldn't be understood that I ended up even worse than usual, slurring my words and speaking much too quickly. In fact, I was rambling and stuttering. Puzzled, my principal said she could not understand what I was saying. She asked me to please repeat what I'd said. With a sigh, I slowed down and tried again.

The same phenomenon began cropping up at home. Whenever I spoke to my husband, he kept asking, "What did you say?" I figured he just hadn't been paying attention the first time. I had to keep repeating myself, which was irritating for both of us and left me feeling tired and frustrated.

Everyone I spoke with thought that they were having a hearing problem, even though I told them I'd lost the power in my voice.

Gradually, I noticed that the daily activities I'd always taken for granted were becoming more and more difficult. I found it hard to hold my food with a fork and cut it. Putting on my socks became an ordeal. It took every ounce of strength just to pull the covers over myself at night, or to push the pillow out from under my head.

I had trouble changing positions in bed or in a car. Sitting at the table for any length of time was unbearable. If I cooked a meal, I was in so much pain that by the time we sat down to eat I was no longer interested. No, that's not so — I'm always interested in eating, I just plain didn't have the strength.

While swimming one day I couldn't maneuver my right leg. It became hard for me to do aerobics in the pool because my toes would have spasms. This was especially mortifying because, in my previous life, I'd been a lifeguard! It was as though life was conspiring to turn all my abilities upside-down. Everything that had once given me pleasure now gave me pain. Driving home after swimming was misery. I felt swealy and shaky. What was happening to me? Was I getting old?

No. This was not normal aging. Something was very wrong.

That autumn, we discovered another possible culprit in my mystery. Some blood work that summer had shown that I had a cholesterol count of 258. My doctor prescribed 10 mg of Lipitor and told me to take a follow-up blood test every month. I don't have good veins and taking blood is always a hassle, so I wasn't quick to go for blood tests on a monthly basis. But I did have my blood checked every once in a while, and my cholesterol count did improve after starting the Lipitor.

I'd been taking Lipitor for a while when I asked my doctor about various aches and pains I hadn't experienced earlier. He told me, "I myself take Lipitor, and I also have muscle aches. You just get used to it."

On November 15, I returned to my primary doctor to complain about my back. I asked him if something was wrong with my lungs or my kidneys. I told him that as the day went on the pain would build up and become more and more unbearable. When I came home from school each night I would begin preparing a salad for supper, but before long would have to stop, take three Advils and lie down. Only when the Advil took effect was I able to finish the salad. That's how I made supper every night. This was not something I could just get used to. But the doctor had no explanation for my symptoms.

One night, I woke from a deep sleep with spasms in my thigh — and it hit me. Maybe it was the Lipitor that was causing the pain in my thigh and back!

I ran down to the office and turned on the computer to do a Google search. I typed in, "Side effects from Lipitor." Sure enough, there it was. One website after another popped up, showing that many people were suffering from the same medication. I printed one of the articles so I could show it to my husband.

> **Lipitor, Neuromuscular Degeneration and Recovery**
>
> Numerous adverse side effect reports have implicated Lipitor and other statin drugs as a probable cause for severe neuromuscular degeneration. Some people who have been using Lipitor for as little as two months report serious muscle weakness and pain. Some who have taken it longer report much more serious symptoms, similar to muscular dystrophy, Parkinson's disease, multiple sclerosis or ALS — Lou Gehrig's disease — in which they are losing neuromuscular control of their bodies or losing significant muscle mass...

I returned to the doctor and told him I was convinced my muscle problems were the result of the Lipitor.

"I don't think it's the Lipitor," he said. "But if you want to run a test, stop the medication for two weeks and then go on it again to see if you feel any worse."

I followed his advice, and noticed that the symptoms were getting worse and worse as time went on. I was convinced it was the Lipitor that was causing my muscle weakness. Or was it muscle damage? Could Lipitor be that harmful? Then and there, I stopped the medication, cold turkey. But a few weeks went by, and my symptoms did not go away.

The doctor suggested that I try prednisone for three days to see if that helped. If it did, he said, I was probably suffering from fibromyalgia. It didn't help. I was back to square one.

No one had answers for me.

In April 2006, we were visiting our friends, Chaim and Chaya Gitty Rosenberg, who live in Monsey. She took one look at me and blurted out, "You look like an old lady! What's wrong with you? You're not walking straight, you're not talking straight, and you don't stop complaining about your muscles. This isn't like you!"

She quickly called her friend Mrs. Radkovsky, who works for Echo, a chesed organization that recommends doctors in the New York-New Jersey area. I had heard of Mrs. Radkovsky from other people she'd helped. In fact, I'd spoken to her on the phone several times myself, when I'd needed a referral to certain specialists. She'd been very helpful in the past, and I'd always wanted to meet her.

Chaya Gitty practically threw me into her car. She drove straight to the Echo office. And then I was standing in front of Mrs. Radkovsky, who studied me intently to see if she could figure out what was wrong with me.

After listening to my story for a few minutes, she wordlessly handed me a list of doctors to call.

I phoned each one, to see if they took my insurance and if there was an appointment available. At each office, the receptionist answered my call with something like,

"Multiple Sclerosis Department, please hold."

I immediately hung up.

Multiple sclerosis! Is that what she thinks I have? Impossible! Doesn't she understand that this is from Lipitor? And that Lipitor can cause muscle problems?

That same month, I was discussing some of my symptoms — particularly, my deteriorating handwriting — with my brother-in-law, Sholom Ginzberg. My script would begin in its regular size and gradually grow smaller and smaller as I wrote. As my hand became more and more tired, my handwriting deteriorated even further, until it became a straight line. My brother-in-law's mouth was agape. He could not read what I had written.

Sholom is a collector of books. Within minutes, he'd sped upstairs to the attic and brought down one of his many medical volumes. He turned to the page that dealt with muscle problems and said, "Read this. Whatever you have sounds serious. Go to a neurologist; don't waste any more time."

I've got to get to the bottom of this before I can't move anymore, I thought to myself. I have to try everything.

I made an appointment to see Dr. Adams in his office, and that is where I found myself on that sunny day in April.

The First Diagnosis

As we waited in Dr. Adams' office, Yossel was handed a clipboard with forms to fill out. I helped him with my medical history and let him deal with the rest. I looked around the waiting room. An old couple was sitting across from us. The man was bent over and quiet. His wife spoke to him, but he didn't respond. He just kept looking around. He seemed confused.

The wife looked at me and smiled. "He has dementia," she said.

"Oh." I couldn't think of anything else to say. I thought about how awful it must be to be that man. And how awful it must be to be his wife. And how embarrassing it must be for her. Was he also embarrassed? I didn't know if people with dementia feel embarrassment. Maybe they do.

I opened the magazine I was holding, but didn't read a word. Yossel completed the forms and returned them. Within minutes, the receptionist called, "Shami Reinman!"

We followed her into a large office with big windows overlooking the street. Dr. Adams was a tall, slender man with sharp features. He came forward and shook Yossel's hand. He must have encountered other orthodox Jewish women in his practice, as he knew not to offer me his hand.

The office had two distinct areas. Directly in front of us was a consultation area, with a large desk, two comfortable chairs facing it and a low bookcase behind. The other part had an examination table and cabinets.

The doctor glanced at the forms Yossel had filled out and invited us to sit. He and Yossel chatted for a minute or two. I could see that my husband liked him. Yossel handed over the MRIs and X-rays, and the doctor perused them for a couple of minutes.

Dr. Adams steepled his fingers and said, "So what brings you here?"

I took a deep breath. "Everything hurts me," I said.

The doctor smiled. "All right, let's get specific. Why don't you start from the beginning? How old are you, Mrs. Reinman?"

"I'm fifty-six years old. My birthday was about two weeks ago."

"And when did your symptoms first appear?"

"It started approximately two years ago."

"So you were about fifty-four years old."

"Yes."

"Tell me about your symptoms."

"Well, my handwriting got worse and worse. We refinanced our house about that time, and there were about a hundred papers to sign. After signing the first few pages, I just couldn't sign my name anymore. My signature was coming out as almost a straight line. And then my voice started getting weaker. My students couldn't hear me."

"What do you teach?"

"Computers and First Aid."

"Interesting. Where do you teach?"

"Ilan High School for Girls in Deal, New Jersey."

"And which grades do you teach?"

"All the grades. I teach Microsoft Word, Illustrator, Excel, Photoshop and InDesign. We even produce our own camera-ready yearbook every year." While I was saying this, it struck me that this was more information than he needed. But he smiled at me kindly.

"I'm sure you're a great teacher," he said. "So you have a computer lab?"

"Yes, we do. I walk around helping the students, but when I have to give instructions to the entire class, I just can't speak loud enough."

"Do you have assistants?"

"I have assistants, but I can't have them do everything. I even invested in my own mike and speakers and installed them in the lab."

"And that helped?"

"A little."

"All right," said the doctor. "Go on. You said that everything was hurting you. What else?"

"It's not really everything, but I'm in so much pain that it seems like it. It started with the big toe on my right foot."

"So what did you do?"

I told him I had seen Dr. Brian Halpern, an orthopedist, who took x-rays and found nothing. I also saw Dr. Lantz, a podiatrist, who injected cortisone directly into the toe but didn't solve the problem. I told him about the pain in my back and the pressure that was pushing my body forward and down.

"And this was all two years ago?" said the doctor.

"Two years ago this coming summer."

"So what happened since then?"

"I was tested for Lyme disease and I took a stress test. Negative. I went to a kinesiologist, but he didn't really help me."

"Well, you're here now." He stood up. "Let's have a look at what's going on. I want you to walk to the far wall and back, placing one foot directly in front of the other."

I found this hard to do. I felt unsteady on my feet, but thought it was probably due to nerves more than anything else. I walked to the wall and turned back. The doctor was watching me intently.

"Now stand still." He came over to stand behind me. "I'm

going to pull you back by the shoulders. Don't worry, I won't let you fall."

I gulped and nodded.

The doctor suddenly took my shoulders and yanked me back quickly. I staggered backward but caught myself before I could fall. I thought that was pretty good.

He placed a footstool next to the examination table. "Do you need help getting onto the table?"

"No," I said, although, considering that I'm a short person, I could have used some help.

He checked my reflexes, and then said that we would do some finger exercises.

"Touch the tip of your index finger to the tip of your thumb," he said, demonstrating with his own fingers. "Touch and let go. Touch and let go. Do it as fast as you can."

He had me do it first with my right hand and then with my left hand. I was able to do it with either hand, but the right hand was definitely slower.

He held up his index finger. "Now touch the tip of my finger with the tip of your index finger and then touch the tip of your nose. As fast as you can."

I managed to do it pretty quickly with either hand, but not quite as fast with my right hand as with my left.

"Now twist your wrists quickly. Palm up, palm down. Palm up, palm down."

Again, my right hand lagged behind.

He put me through several similar exercises. Then we went to sit at his desk.

The doctor handed me a piece of paper and a pen. "Please write a sentence."

I started writing something, but as I wrote, the letters kept getting smaller and smaller until they dissolved into hardly more than a straight line. The doctor took the paper and studied it for a moment. Then he put it aside.

"So what's the verdict?" asked Yossel.

The doctor turned to me. "Before I say anything, I want to know what you think is wrong with you."

"I have a little hypoglycemia. Maybe that's causing it."

"Hypoglycemia didn't cause those symptoms."

"Maybe it's Lipitor."

The doctor shook his head. "It's not Lipitor."

"I don't know," I said. "I think maybe I had a small stroke. I think it's something serious ... more serious than I thought."

The doctor looked me straight in the eye. "You have Parkinson's disease."

Although I was prepared for bad news, the doctor's words hit me with a stunning blow. I couldn't believe it.

But deep down, I did.

I'd known for a long time that something was terribly wrong. Little by little, my body had turned on me until it felt like an enemy instead of a friend. It just never occurred to me that it was Parkinson's.

I looked at Yossel. His jaw had dropped open in deep shock. Optimist that he was, he was totally unprepared for such bad news.

For a minute or so, no one spoke. The doctor's words hung in the room like a dark cloud. Then Yossel spoke. I heard him through a haze.

"So what can we do about it?" he asked.

"There are things we can do to make you better," the doctor said, looking at me. "You are only fifty-six years old. That's very young for Parkinson's. Usually, we see it in people seventy or older. But we can help you with medication."

"If I'm too young for this," I said, "are you sure that's what it is?"

"Yes, I'm sure. I see many, many Parkinson's patients, and I can recognize it when I see it."

"But how can you tell?" I persisted. "I thought I did pretty well on the tests."

"Your posture is not good. You walk with a stoop, leaning forward. Your right arm doesn't swing by your side when you walk. Your handwriting is a dead giveaway. The letters get very tiny, until they're just a line. You have micrographia. It's a sure sign of Parkinson's."

"So you're sure?"

"I'm sure."

By this time, Yossel had recovered a little. His jaw wasn't hanging open any more.

"So where do we go from here, doctor?" he asked. "I understand that Parkinson's is a degenerative disease."

"We like to call it a progressive disease."

"Which means the same thing."

The doctor nodded. "Yes, it does. The disease progresses over time, and function diminishes."

"What are you saying?" I said. "Is this it? It's terrible now, and it's just going to get worse and worse?" Much as I dreaded his answer, I needed to hear it. Not knowing, the lack of clarity that I'd been struggling with as my symptoms worsened over the months, was almost worse than anything he might say.

The doctor shook his head. "Your life is not over, Mrs. Reinman. With medication, we can make you almost one hundred percent better. Don't worry. This is not a death sentence. You can have a normal life for many years to come. Your brain is not producing enough dopamine, so messages from your brain to your body travel more slowly, and your movements are affected. But we can compensate. I'll prescribe medication for you. It's Stalevo, with Compton and Selegeline. You have to build up the medicine in your system gradually. Don't take any more than I prescribe for you.

"I'm also going to give you a prescription for an MRI of your brain, to rule out multiple sclerosis or a brain tumor. I don't think you have either of those, but just to be on the safe side, let's make sure."

He stood up, and so did we.

"You'll be fine, Mrs. Reinman," he said as he walked us to the door. "We'll take good care of you."

Outside, the sun was still shining, and the sky was still blue. But I was in a daze. It was as if a heavy door had slammed shut behind me, separating the Shami I was now, this minute, to the one who'd walked out of the car an hour before. Compared to the way I felt now, the apprehension I'd felt on the way to this appointment seemed, in retrospect, like a carefree run in the park. I looked at Yossel, and I could see him making an effort to be positive.

"It's going to be okay, Shami," he told me. "You heard what the doctor said. He can make you one hundred percent better."

I gave him a sickly smile. "He didn't say he can make me one hundred percent well. He said he can make me one hundred percent better than I am now. That's not the same thing. It's still pretty bad."

"It's still something," he said.

My Grandmother Suspects

On Sunday, I went to visit my maternal grandmother in the Boro Park section of Brooklyn, as I'd been doing every week for over twenty years.

My grandmother was a very great, very wise and very holy woman. She passed away in the summer of 2007, at the age of one hundred and five, and was sharp as a knife until the last few months of her life. Her great-grandchildren called her Bobby Ima, to differentiate her from their grandmothers. She was the queen of our family in every way.

Bobby Ima was much more than a grandmother to me, and to all of us. She was our connection to our illustrious ancestors, not only because she knew them and told us stories about them, but even more because she herself was one of them. She was our bridge to a Jewish world that was simpler, purer and holier than the one in which we lived.

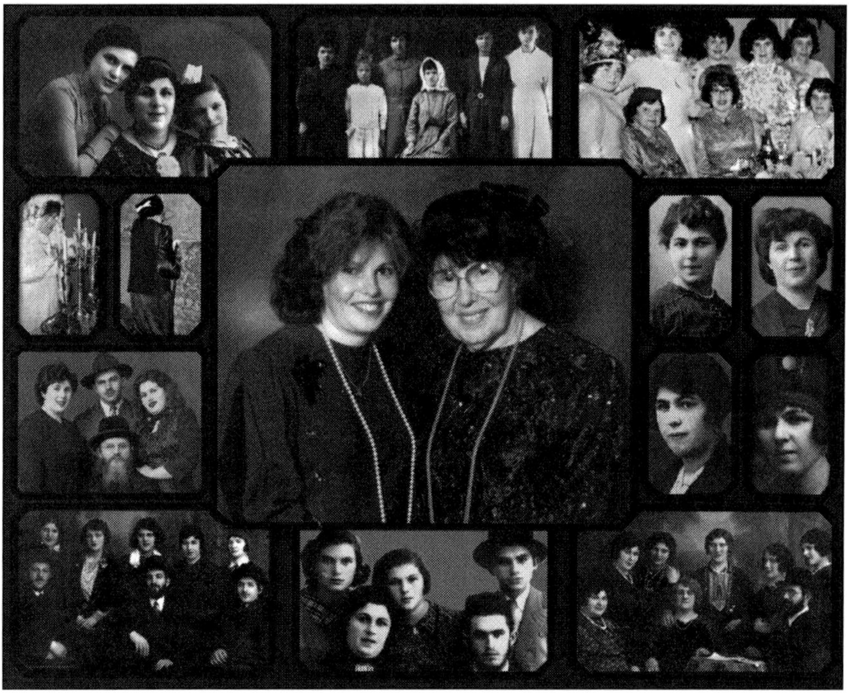

Collage of Bobby Ima. Pictured centered top is Bobbe Shlomtza, Bobby Ima's mother-in-law, the author's namesake. Collage prepared by the author.

Through her, we felt connected to earlier generations, which made us feel proud and privileged but also placed a heavy sense of responsibility on our shoulders. She was our role model, and through her, our ancestors also became our role models as well. Speaking for myself, I felt that I had to measure up to them at least a little bit .

My mother's father, Rav Yissachar Ber Shapiro, was the Kechnier Rebbe, a direct descendant of Rav Pinchas of Koritz and a great-grandson of Rav Sholom Mordechai Schwadron, the Berzhaner Rav, known as the Maharsham. My mother's mother, Rechel Rosenbaum, known in our family as Bobby Ima, was the daughter of Rav Isamar Rosenbaum, the Nadvorner Rebbe and a grandson of Rav Mordche of Nadvorna. Rav Isamar's sister Shlomtza, my namesake, was my grandfather's mother, which made my grandparents first cousins.

When the time came for me to start *shidduchim,* my parents

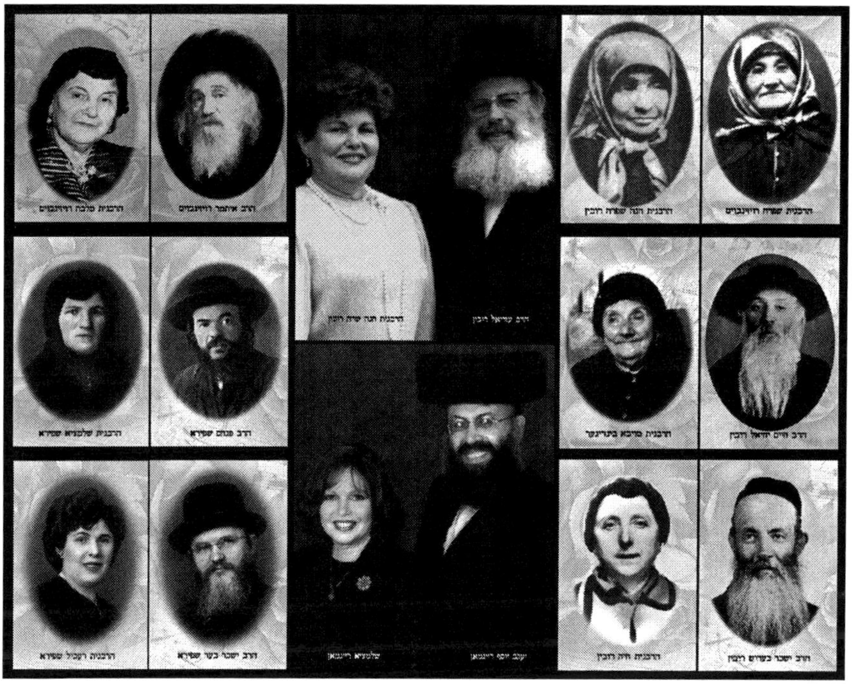

Collage of the author's family. Collage prepared by the author.

would first seek the approval of Bobby Ima's father, my great-grandfather, whom we called Zeidiku. One after another, Zeidiku turned them down. But when Yossel's name came up, Zeidiku said, "Reinman is a good name. You should look into it."

Of course, Yossel had more than just a good family going for him. He was brilliant, a rising star, one of the best boys in the Lakewood Yeshivah. That was much more important to me than his lineage. In any case, Yossel was the first and only boy I dated. Yossel claims I didn't marry him because I liked him but because Zeidiku basically ordered me to. But he's only joking. He knows that isn't true.

I adored Zeidiku. He had a shul in Washington Heights, and we didn't see him that often, only on Chanukah and Purim. All the grandchildren would come to watch him light the *menorah* and to bring him *mishloach manos*. He would sit in his huge armchair and sing old Nadvorner songs while he played the fiddle. When he smiled at me and called me Shlomtza Kapomtza, my young heart would swell with joy and pride.

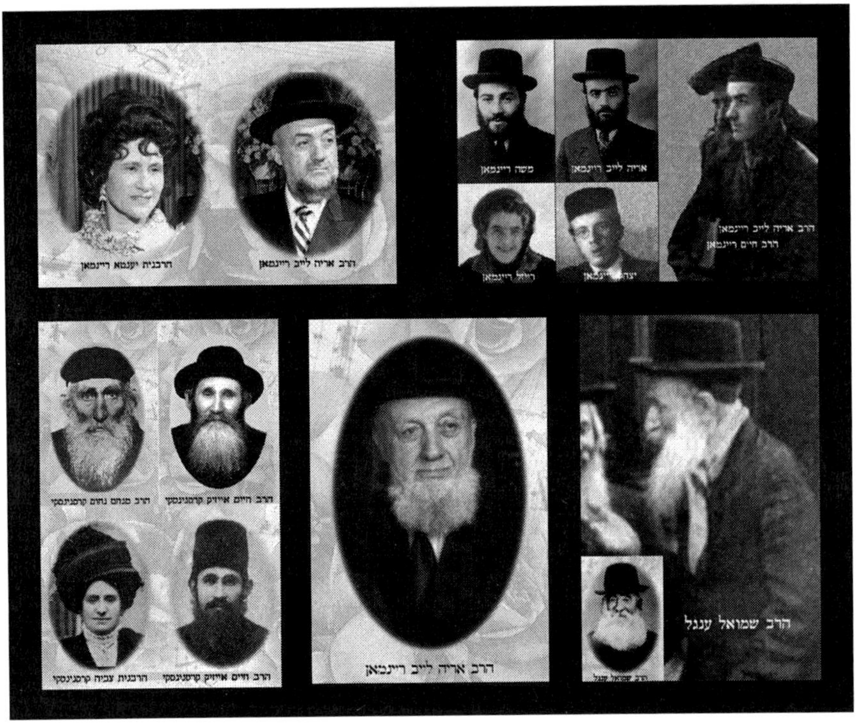

Collage of the author's husband's family. Collage prepared by the author.

My great-grandmother, Zeidiku's wife, was Bobbe Malka. We called her Bobbiku. She was the daughter of Rav Asher Yeshayah Rubin of Kolbysov, a descendant of the Ropschitz dynasty and a distant cousin of my father's. Bobbiku was five years older than Zeidiku and always seemed quite ancient to me, not nearly as strong and vigorous as Zeidiku was. She was very good at chess and loved to play. Like all good chess players, she took the game very seriously. She used to smile at me and kiss me, but other than that she didn't give me much attention. I was just one of over a hundred great-grandchildren. I loved Bobbiku, but I adored Zeidiku.

I always hoped that Zeidiku would live to come to my wedding. Bobbiku had passed away several years before I married, but Zeidiku was still alive and well. Then, just six months before my wedding, at the ripe old age of eighty-four, my great-grandfather decided to pick himself up from Washington Heights and open a shul in the Yad Eliyahu section of Tel Aviv. I was terribly upset. But two months after we were married, we went to Eretz Yisrael for ten weeks and spent a lot of time with Zeidiku. He and Yossel really hit it off. They would talk together for hours, and I enjoyed sitting and watching them.

Bobby Ima told me many stories about Zeidiku as a young man. She told me about his father, Rav Meyer Kretchniver, and his grandfather, Rav Mordche Nadvorner. She loved to tell one story in particular. I heard it from her many times. She never tired of telling it.

Zeidiku was all of fourteen years old when he married Bobbiku. She was nineteen. After their wedding, they lived in Kolbysov, Poland, in the home of Bobbiku's parents, who supported the young couple while Zeidiku continued studying. But Zeidiku was an independent young man who didn't relish living under the thumb of his wife's parents. One year later, when Bobby Ima was still a newborn, Zeidiku decided to move on. He'd heard good things about the Jewish community in Czernowitz, Romania, hundreds of miles away, and after making some inquiries, he felt there was an opportunity for him there. He would open a shul in Czernowitz, and following in the footsteps of his father and grandfathers, he would become a Rebbe in his own right.

In 1902, when he was just turning sixteen, he left his wife and infant daughter in Kolbysov and traveled to Czernowitz. A very talented and charismatic young man, he managed to attract a group of followers. Within two months, he opened his shul. Then he sent a telegram to his wife, asking her to join him.

There were no high-speed trains in those days. The train from Kolbysov stopped in many towns and cities along the way to Czernowitz. The three-day journey was a difficult one for Bobbiku, traveling on her own with many packages and valises and a baby in her arms. The baby was running a fever and crying hysterically when the station master shouted for Bobbiku and the other passengers to board the train. In the commotion, she left some of her belongings on the platform.

A few stops later, when the baby had calmed down a bit, she checked her baggage and realized that a number of valises were missing. She was beside herself. Everything she owned in the world was in that baggage — and now, a good part of it was gone. What was she going to do?

At the next stop, a young man got onto the train and came over to her. He had brought the rest of her baggage. Clutching her crying baby, she thanked him profusely. The young man sat across from her and took the child from her aching arms. He managed to calm the baby, who soon fell asleep. In this way, he accompanied Bobbiku all the way to Czernowitz, holding the baby in his arms most of the time. He reassured Bobbiku that the baby would be fine and that she needn't worry.

When they arrived at the station in Czernowitz, Zeidiku and a group of his followers were waiting to greet the new arrivals. Bobbiku told Zeidiku about the young man who had been such a lifesaver during the difficult journey. Zeidiku, wanting to thank him, searched high and low, but the young man was nowhere to be found. Bobby Ima — the baby in the episode — told me many years later that Zeidiku and Bobbiku were convinced that the young man was Eliyahu Hanavi, sent by Heaven to help her. It was a beautiful story, and I loved hearing it every time she repeated it to me or to my children.

At other times, Bobby Ima told me about her childhood. Czernowitz was a modern city, and raising a Chassidic family there was not easy. Zeidiku kept his children at home most of the time. He hired a *melamed*, a tutor of Jewish studies, to learn with his sons, but the boys were not eager to spend so many hours cooped up in the house. One day, Bobby Ima came back from the market to find some of her brothers sitting on the stoop, holding bundles in their laps and crying.

"What's going on?" she asked in astonishment.

"We weren't learning," they said through a river of tears, "so *der Totte* packed these bundles of our things and sent us out. He said we were on our own and could go wherever we want, but we can't stay here anymore."

"Don't cry," she told them. "If you promise to pay more attention to your learning, I'll talk to *der Totte* and ask him to let you back in."

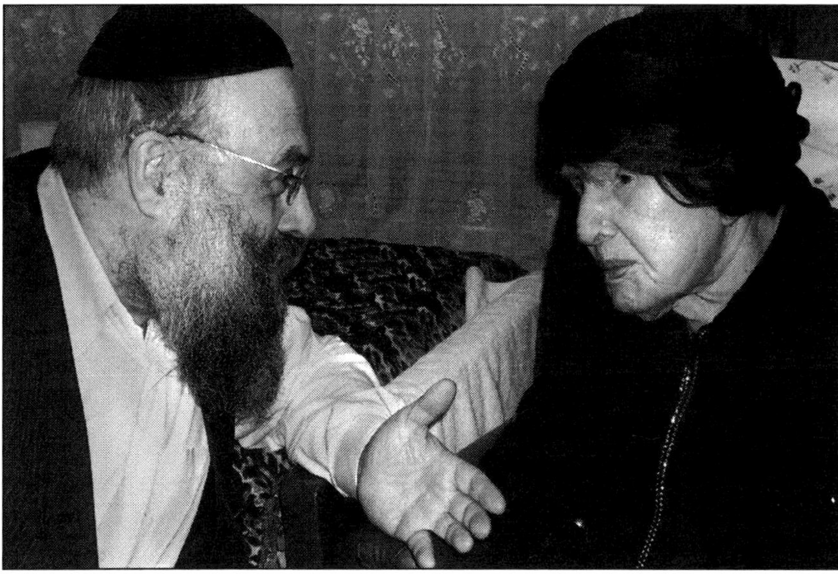

The author's husband and Bobby Ima

Her brothers gladly agreed. There was no more trouble with the *melamed* after that.

There was no *melamed* for Bobby Ima. She had her hands full helping her mother run the household. Still, she managed to listen in on her brothers' sessions and became very knowledgeable. She always had an unquenchable thirst for knowledge, a quick brain and a pure spirit. Zeidiku would say that if she had been a boy she would have made an excellent Rebbe.

Bobby Ima and Yossel liked and respected each other. She was very proud of him, and he valued her opinions. She was his grandmother by marriage for thirty-seven years, and the two were as close as if she'd been his natural grandmother .

A year or two before she passed away, Yossel asked her, "How did you merit such a long life?" This is a question the rabbis in the Talmud sometimes asked very old people.

"How should I know?" she said. "Am I a *neviah* (prophetess) or something?"

Then, a minute later, she gave him an answer.

"I was always a very good daughter to my parents," she said. "In my whole life, I never made them angry or upset."

That's pretty amazing. I can't say the same about myself. Actually, I don't know anyone who can.

Bobby Ima also told me many stories about her marriage, and about how she and my grandfather ended up in America before the Second World War and managed to rescue the remnants of the family. Most of all, I pressed her for stories about Bobbe Shlomtza, her mother-in-law and aunt, whose name I carry. Both Bobbe Shlomtza and my great-grandfather were murdered in the Holocaust. I had a few pictures of her, but I wanted to know what she was like. I wanted to know if I had any of her in me.

Bobby Ima told me that Bobbe Shlomtza was a wonderful woman, with an exceptionally kind heart. When she was a little girl, she had only two dresses, one for weekdays and another for Shabbos. One day, her mother bought her a new Shabbos dress, and Shlomtza was very excited. As she stood in front of the mirror, admiring herself in her new dress, her father called her over.

"Shlomtza, you know that little girl across the street," he said. "Her family is very poor, and she doesn't have a Shabbos dress. How would you like to give her that dress? It would make her very happy."

"Of course," she said immediately, with a smile. She slipped off the new dress, went across the street and gave it to their poor neighbor.

I'm sure she was sad that she would not have a new dress, after all. But at the same time, the real pleasure she derived from making a poor little girl happy made up for it.

I like to think that I, too, have a good heart and a generous nature. I used to give my clothes to one of my cousins, even though they still fit. In fact, she was much taller than I was and actually had to add material so that she could wear them. I always felt good about that. In summer camp, quite a few girls were wearing my clothes, and I didn't mind one bit.

When the Germans came to Kechnia, they deported Rav Pinchas, my great-grandfather, and Bobbe Shlomtza, my great-grandmother, to Auschwitz. They were both sent to the left side in the selection as soon as they were driven from the cattle cars.

On that same day, they were murdered in the gas chambers, and their bodies were burned in the crematoria.

Bobbe Shlomtza was Zeidiku's sister. If she'd survived, I would have grown up knowing her, just as I knew Zeidiku, who passed away in 1973. I know I would have been close to her. What a tremendous, senseless loss. Those murderers left an empty place in my life, and in my heart.

My grandfather's youngest sister, Bobbe Shlomtza's daughter, was my great-aunt Shifrah, the Kalever Rebbetzin of Yerushalayim. She was the wife of Rav Menachem Mendel Taub, the renowned Kalever Rebbe. They were married in 1944, right before the Germans invaded Hungary, and were separated from each other until the war was over. My great-aunt had many stories to tell about their experiences. After the war, they lived for a time in the United States, first in Cleveland, Ohio and then in the Bensonhurst section of Brooklyn, N.Y.

Growing up, I was very close to my aunt, and we remained close during all the years afterward. Whenever Yossel and I went to Eretz Yisrael, we often stayed with them for part of the time. In 1995, when our son Berel went to study in a yeshivah in Eretz Yisrael, he didn't want to come home for Pesach. He was very involved in his learning and felt that coming home would break the momentum. Instead, he wanted us to come to Eretz Yisrael to be with him. On the other hand, our daughter Devora and son Chaim, who were already married, didn't want us to go away for Pesach, which was a Yom Tov they'd expected to share with us at home.

Unable to resolve the dilemma, we asked Bobby Ima for advice. She told us that this was a critical time in Berel's development, and that we should go to him instead of tearing him away from the yeshivah. So we went. We spent the first days with my son-in-law Tzvi's brother, Aharon Follman, and his family in Har Nof, and the second days in Bnei Brak with the Kalever Rebbe and Rebbetzin. It was a very precious time for me, because I was able to spend many, many hours talking with my aunt. I especially wanted to know about her mother, my great-grandmother, Bobbe Shlomtza.

The Kalever Rebbetzin was very happy to have someone with whom to converse at such great length about her childhood and her parents — especially someone who was deeply interested and cared so much.

Rav Pinchas, her father and my great-grandfather, was the rabbi of Kechnia and also a Chassidic Rebbe. He was an outstanding Torah scholar and wrote a *sefer* called *Tzafnas Paanayach*. The Maharsham, his mother's father, was very proud of him. When Rav Pinchas decided to become a Rebbe, the Maharsham gave him his first *kvittel*. He used to recite the entire *Tehillim* every morning before Shacharis, and then spent almost the entire rest of the day studying his holy volumes.

Rav Pinchas opened his home to every traveler and poor person, and it was his wife, my Bobbe Shlomtza, who took care of them. Every evening in their home, the Kalever Rebbetzin told me, Bobbe Shlomtza prepared supper for over one hundred people. From her earliest memories as a little girl, the Kalever Rebbetzin remembered spending all day, every day, helping her mother prepare the food. The meals were simple but always more than enough to fill all those hungry bellies. And when Bobbe Shlomtza had a little spare time, she sat in a corner and recited *Tehillim*.

One day, she was preparing a chicken when she suddenly shrank back. She went to her husband and told him, "We can't eat that chicken. It's not kosher."

"How do you know?" he asked. "It came from a reliable kosher butcher. Why do you suspect there is something wrong with it?"

"I don't know. I just have a feeling."

It was no simple thing to throw away a chicken because of a suspicion based on a feeling. Nonetheless, her husband did not take her words lightly. He called for the butcher and questioned him. Based on what he heard, he realized that the chicken was indeed questionable at best.

That was my Bobbe Shlomtza.

The Kalever Rebbetzin could not tell me much about my grandfather. He was much older and was married and living in another town while she was growing up.

My grandfather married Bobby Ima right after the First World War. She was almost seventeen years old. He was not much older. They settled in the small town of Novosellitz, Romania, where he was offered the position of rabbi. The years in Novosellitz were good. They had two boys and two girls. My mother, Chanah Sarah, was the youngest. They had everything they needed. They even had their own cow. My grandfather was happy, but Bobby Ima wasn't. There was no yeshivah in Novosellitz for her sons, and although they hired a *melamed* for them, Bobby Ima felt that her boys were losing out. She wanted to move to a larger town.

One day, Bobby Ima heard that their great-uncle by marriage, the Shtefaneshter Rebbe, a very elderly sage renowned for his wisdom and holiness, was visiting a nearby town, and she prevailed upon her husband to seek his advice.

The Rebbe listened quietly as they presented their arguments. Then he closed his eyes and thought for a while. "I don't see anything else for you here in Romania," he said at last.

My grandfather felt that he had been vindicated, and they returned to Novosellitz. Several months later, the Shtefaneshter Rebbe passed away.

A few days after his passing, the Rebbe came to my grandfather in a dream. "I told you that I see nothing for you and your family here in Romania," he said. "Or anywhere else in Europe. Go to Eretz Yisrael as soon as you can. As for reaching Eretz Yisrael, it will be difficult, but you will succeed. I will help you."

My grandfather was shaken by the dream, and they immediately began preparations for the emigration, to the dismay of their parents and siblings. It was almost unheard of for young couples in their circles to make such a move, to separate from their families and undertake the hardships of the journey and life in Eretz Yisrael, then known as Palestine. It was 1937, and Palestine was in the hands of the British. The doors were firmly closed to Jewish immigration, and except for the very well-connected, it was almost impossible to obtain immigration certificates. But my grandmother persevered. My husband always says that I'm the most tenacious person he knows. I guess I take after Bobby Ima in that, at least.

My grandfather wrote a letter to Rav Kook asking him to help him obtain certificates for his family. He had absolutely no connection to Rav Kook, but he decided to try anyway. Amazingly, a short while later, a letter arrived from Rav Kook accompanied by certificates for the family. It was practically miraculous, and my grandparents were convinced that it could only be attributed to the efforts of the Shtefaneshter Rebbe in *Shamayim*.

The old Rebbe had also told my grandfather that it would be difficult to make the move, and indeed it was. Eretz Yisrael did not turn out to be the paradise they had envisioned, but they were not murdered by the Nazis as were many of the family members they'd left behind. They were penniless and literally starving, but the boys went to good yeshivahs and were doing well, which made Bobby Ima very happy. The bright future that beckoned for them, however, was not in Eretz Yisrael but in America. In 1939, my grandfather left for New York to make arrangements to bring his family there.

After several brutal years in Eretz Yisrael, the family followed my grandfather to America and settled in the Lower East Side. A few years later, my grandparents bought a house in the Bronx with borrowed money and opened a shul. During and after the war years, my grandparents worked day and night to bring family members from blood-soaked Europe to safety and a new life in America. Bobby Ima met with Irving Bunim and enlisted his help in obtaining visas for her relatives. Each visa cost about five hundred dollars. Since my grandparents had no money, they borrowed thousands of dollars to pay for the precious visas. They spent many years paying back these loans, in addition to the loans they'd taken out to buy the house.

My grandfather passed away in 1954, at the age of 57, when I was just four years old. My memories of him are vague. I probably would not remember him at all, if it weren't for an old home movie that's lasted down the years. Yossel's father told me that he knew my grandfather and that he was a very nice person. I seem to remember him being nice, but I'm not sure if it's a real memory.

The movie was taken a few months before he passed away, when he was already very sick. In the movie, he is lighting the Chanukah candles, and the family is watching him with sad eyes. Then I come into view: a cute little girl playing a flute, oblivious to anything that might be going on around me.

After my grandfather passed away, my grandmother ran the shul for many years, and for most of my childhood that shul became one of the focal points of my life. Our family went there often for Shabbos, so that my father could help out in the shul. And the whole extended family regularly descended on the Bronx to spend the holidays at Bobby Ima's house.

On Chanukah, Bobby Ima lit the candles and said the blessings, while everyone watched and listened. Then she distributed dollar bills to all of her grandchildren. If she suspected that a granddaughter was expecting a child, she asked how many dollars she needed. I still have several of those dollar bills.

On the eight-day festivals of Pesach and Succos, all of us packed into her house again. We kids slept on the floor, but we didn't mind. We were together with all of our cousins, and we had a wonderful time. On Succos, the men ate in the *succah* while the women had their meals in the house. Except for Bobby Ima. All her life, until the very last months, when she was practically on her deathbed, she never took as much as a sip of water outside of the *succah*.

Thinking back on those times, I realize how hard my grandmother must have worked to pull off those family get-togethers, but she didn't complain. She'd been raised to work hard, and she enjoyed an ongoing conversation with the Almighty as she worked.

A few years before I was married, Bobby Ima sold the house in the Bronx to the Navy and moved to an apartment in Boro Park, where the family could visit her more often. She lived on her own, though she frequently came to our house for Shabbos meals. She lit many candles for Shabbos — so many I could barely count them — and she always made her own *Kiddush*. On Shabbos afternoons she would recite the entire *Tehillim* and then accept the stream of visitors that came to see her. But she'd been having problems with her knees for a long time. It became more and more difficult for her to walk. And she was getting older.

In 1978, when my parents built a house on Fifty-Eighth Street in Boro Park, they set aside part of the first floor as a private apartment for Bobby Ima. She lived there for the rest of her life, even after both of my parents passed away.

It was not easy for my mother to have her mother living downstairs. My mother was a special person, but she could not compare or compete with her mother, who was a major star. Bobby Ima was like a gentle queen, holding court at her dining-room table. Grandchildren, other relatives and friends came to visit her all the time. Whenever I came, there was always a tug-of-war between my mother and grandmother for my time. In the end, we decided to alternate weeks. When it was my mother's week, I just popped in to say hello to Bobby Ima and then went upstairs to visit my mother.

After she turned eighty, we grandchildren realized that she was going to be more or less homebound. We decided to establish a rotation of visitors to make sure she had company every day. Apart from traveling in weekly from Lakewood to visit her, I undertook the responsibility of maintaining the rotation calendar. It was a major task, and I did it for twenty years.

Today, I find myself in a similar situation. I am homebound, and my good friend Bayla Stein has taken charge of the calendar so that I have at least one or two visitors every day. Because it's hard for me to speak, we spend most of our time playing Upwords. But more about that later. Being in this situation myself, I realize how much my efforts meant to Bobby Ima, and consider it a privilege to have been able to do that for her.

As she aged, her body began to break down. Her eyesight and hearing deteriorated. I made enlarged copies of the Siddur, which she found very useful, but she didn't like using hearing aids. Her knees were giving way. In 1986, at the age of eighty-five, she decided she wanted knee-replacement surgery. Family members tried to dissuade her from having major surgery at her age, but she was determined.

"Do you expect me to be in a wheelchair for the rest of my life?" she said. "I want to walk." She knew that artificial knees last for ten years, and she wanted those ten additional years of walking.

So she checked herself into the Hospital for Special Surgery in Manhattan and had her knees fixed. Yossel and I sent our children to relatives for Shabbos and spent Shabbos in the hospital with her. On Shabbos morning, Yossel walked to Rabbi David Bleich's shul on East Seventy-Eighth Street, wearing his fur *shtreimel*. On his return, he reported that many people had turned to stare at him. "They probably don't see a *shtreimel* very often on the Upper East Side," he remarked. "I don't mind if they stare, as long as they don't hit."

Ten years later, the new knee gave out. Bobby Ima, now ninety-five years old, decided to have her knee replaced again, this time in Lennox Hill Hospital in Manhattan. By then, Yossel's cousin, Rabbi Benzion Krasniansky, had opened a Chabad house on the Upper East Side, and we stayed with them for Shabbos and spent many hours in the hospital with Bobby Ima.

On that Sunday in April, 2006, just a few days after I'd learned the nature of my affliction, I visited Bobby Ima as I did every week. I was a wreck. All my life, I'd known that in times of trouble I could turn to my parents and to Bobby Ima. But my parents were no longer alive. My mother had passed away in 2000, and my father in 2005. My husband was not the answer. He was in the same boat as I was, equally devastated. The only one left was Bobby Ima. I could always count on her to provide strength and encouragement. But she was now one hundred and four years old, a shadow of her former self.

I came into the room and found her asleep in her bed, barely breathing. She opened her eyes and looked up at me with her sightless eyes. All she could make out were shapes, and possibly colors.

"Shami, is that you?" she asked.

"Yes, Bobby, it's me. How are you?"

She didn't answer right away. I could see her straining and thinking.

"Are you all right, darling?" she finally said. Maybe she heard something in my voice. Maybe she read my body language. I don't know how she sensed my distress.

At that moment, I decided not to burden her with my troubles. She was weak and in constant pain, hanging on to life by a thread. She didn't need me to dump a huge burden in her lap. All it would accomplish would be to cause her anguish and anxiety.

"I'm fine, Bobby," I said.

"You don't sound fine, mamaleh. What's the matter?"

"Nothing, Bobby. I'm fine. Really."

"You don't want to tell me," she said. With a sigh, she closed her eyes and drifted back to sleep.

Side Effects

Doctor Adams was certain that it was Parkinson's disease. On one level, buried deep, I accepted the truth of his diagnosis. I'd already enlisted the help of a wide variety of physicians and specialists to try and make sense of the clues, but all their theories had hit a dead end. Here was a diagnosis that seemed consistent with all my symptoms.

But on another, more conscious level, I refused to be convinced. An earthquake may have shaken my life, but I was simply not prepared to let the earth swallow me up. I wasn't ready to give up my life as I knew it, my activities, taking care of my family, my teaching, my traveling, my freedom of movement. I wasn't ready to become an invalid!

Nonetheless, I did begin taking the pills he prescribed. I was supposed to build up to the prescribed dosage over a period of three weeks, to make sure I could tolerate the medication. This made me nervous. What kind of powerful drugs was I introducing into my body?

On the other hand, what else could I do? Passive suffering made no sense. I could only take the pills, and hope that I'd eventually find someone who would give me a better diagnosis.

So I took my medicine.

And then came the side effects.

A neighbor of mine had just married off a child, and the neighbors on our block were making *sheva berachos* in honor of the new couple. The thought of sitting home and brooding about my health was unappealing, so I dressed up and went across the street to attend.

It was a disaster. My arms were so weak that I had trouble getting the fork from my plate to my mouth. The more I tried, the more nervous I became. Finally, I gave up and decided to go home. The hostess walked me to the door and asked if I was feeling okay.

"I've been better," I said briefly and made my escape.

The next morning, as I was brushing my teeth, I looked into the mirror and noticed something very odd and even comical. I was nodding my head up and down to brush my teeth, instead of using the up-and-down motion of my right hand as I normally did.

I went out and bought an electric toothbrush.

Dr. Adams had prescribed physical therapy for me, so I started attending a group practice in the town of Long Branch, New Jersey. One of the therapists noticed that my eyeballs were moving behind my lids when I closed my eyes. She told me that this was not supposed to happen with Parkinson's, and suggested that I might have something else.

With a flash of hope, I asked her what she thought it was. She didn't know, but she gave me the name of a local neurologist whom she highly recommended. The neurologist's name was Dr. Vicky Rabb. Her office was on Route 35 in Deal. We made an appointment, and Yossel and I went to see her.

Dr. Rabb was a tall woman with short, dark hair. She was kind, gracious and sensitive, and she made me realize how much more comfortable I felt with a woman doctor. She administered a battery of tests similar to those Dr. Adams had given me. I was told to touch my fingers to my nose, open and close my hands quickly, and so on.

And then came the verdict. Parkinson's.

Clutching at straws, I asked if the trouble I was having with my arms could be carpal tunnel syndrome. Obligingly, she had me tested for it. The test was very painful, and it came back negative. There was no denying the results so far: My symptoms were all Parkinsonian.

I still wasn't satisfied. Dr. Adams and Dr. Rabb were general neurologists. They also dealt with other conditions: epilepsy, cerebral palsy, stroke and other problems related to the nervous system. I wanted to hear the diagnosis from a top specialist in Parkinson's disease. Though I knew it was true, I wasn't ready to admit it yet. And if I did turn out to have that condition, I definitely wanted to be under the care of a top Parkinson's specialist. We needed to find one in the New York area.

We called everyone we could think of, and then expanded our search by contacting community activists with an expertise in medical referrals. These included Mrs. Miriam Lubling, as well as Rabbi Shuky Berman and Mrs. Radkowsky of ECHO in Monsey, New York. ECHO recommended Dr. Cheryl Waters, Dr. Blair Ford and Dr. Lucian Coté, all of whom practiced in Columbia Presbyterian. Rabbi Berman said that Dr. Stanley Fahn, also in Columbia, was probably the best doctor in the field, but he had no connection in that office and could not help us get an appointment. He also recommended Dr. Susan Bressman of Beth Israel Medical Center and Dr. Warren Olanow of Mount Sinai Medical Center. I really wanted a woman doctor, and decided to go with Dr. Bressman because I'd heard that she was a warm and caring person.

Then came the great appointment struggle.

All these doctors are in great demand, and their calendars are full. Here we were in June, and the first opening was way off in January. Rabbi Berman made a few calls. My husband also called many, many times and wrote letters.

Eventually, we were given an appointment in October 2006. We were satisfied with that. There really wasn't any emergency. I was taking the medications Dr. Adams had prescribed for me, and they were helping a little. And at least I had the peace of mind of knowing that I'd been accepted as Dr. Bressman's patient.

It had been a difficult spring. Behind everything I did was the knowledge that I'd been handed a harsh sentence, and it was called PD. I was still teaching, still trying my best to stay fit. Shortly after my visit to Dr. Adams, I lost my balance for the first time.

It happened in an aerobics class in the gym. We were doing an exercise dance, when I suddenly found myself falling backward. I staggered back five steps before I was able to catch myself and regain my balance. It was the scariest feeling: I had lost control of my body for a few seconds. I sat down and waited for my heart to stop pounding. Then I went home.

One morning, I woke up to find my pillow soaking wet. To my horror, I realized that I was drooling. Some nights, I screamed in my sleep. The screams were so loud that they woke my husband. Yossel is a sound sleeper, so I must have been really loud. To get me to stop, he had to wake me. Sometimes, the screams came from nightmares about losing my balance and falling. I slept so deeply that whatever was on my mind that day came to the surface and erupted out of my throat. I would wake in the morning with my elbow crooked and my hand bent forward under my chin, ice-cold from lack of circulation.

The situations were mounting. One night, I woke up with a terrible toothache. It was too early to call the dentist, so I took some Advil for the pain and went into the kitchen to distract myself with some cooking. By 9:00 a.m. I was sitting in the dentist's chair.

I'd been having trouble brushing my teeth, but this pain was simply unbearable. Dr. Wasserman placed cold cotton gauze on every tooth to see where the pain was coming from, but he couldn't pinpoint it.

Finally, he sent me to a root-canal specialist in Monmouth. He arranged a three o'clock appointment on Friday afternoon. Luckily, thanks to my early cooking, most of my Shabbos food was prepared.

The dental specialist took me in right away. He used the same method as Dr. Wasserman, except that his method was more intense. He made each tooth painfully cold and then checked my jaws and my gums. Each time he pressed on my gums, I screamed.

"Maybe you are having muscle spasms or TMJ," he said. "Do you grind your teeth at night or press them tightly together?"

"Yes, I press my teeth together at night," I told him. "I've been very nervous lately, because I have just been diagnosed with PD."

He looked at me with a mix of surprise and pity and said, "You're too young. It can't be."

But I knew that it was. The dentist didn't charge anything. When we said good-bye, he wished me luck. I appreciated his help, and his good wishes.

At school the next morning, Frumie Feller, a colleague and very close friend of mine, came over with a soft, concerned expression and asked me how I was feeling.

That was all I needed. I could barely speak through the tears.

"What's wrong, Shami?" she asked in alarm.

"I just found out I have Parkinson's disease!"

We hugged and cried together. It's amazing how much comfort there can be in a simple human outpouring of love and sympathy. I might not have had the full use of my once-vigorous body, but I definitely had a friend.

When we'd calmed down enough to face the world again, both of us went to teach our classes. I wondered if I should have just skipped school that day. But what good would it do to sit home and mope?

That policy seemed to sum up my life right then. Try to keep functioning normally. Until I hit a brick wall. One step forward and another step back. Fall apart emotionally, but keep on going.

Always keep on going.

Travel Plans

Yossel really likes to travel, and I enjoy it, too. We've been to Eretz Yisrael many times, as well as many other places. Since we couldn't see Dr. Bressman until October and there was nothing holding us at home, he wanted to take a trip. A granddaughter of my great-aunt, the Kalever Rebbetzin, was to be married in Eretz Yisrael in late August, and I suggested that we attend the wedding.

Yossel didn't go for that idea; he had a desire to visit Spain, Venice and Switzerland.

"Three countries will definitely be too much for me," I told him regretfully. "I could fly to one of them with you, and then continue on to Eretz Yisrael myself."

After I'd convinced him that this plan made the most sense in light of my condition, I urged, "Choose the place that we'll visit together."

My husband never hesitated. "Spain," he said.

Why Spain?

This is the story.

When Yossel and I were married, he was learning in yeshivah full-time. We were for the most part supported by my father, who was a successful diamond dealer, though I also worked. I was a teacher in a Hebrew school, and at night my friend Mirel Simcha and I strung gold links into chains until our fingertips were sore. Then an opportunity came along for me to teach at Bais Kaila High School in Lakewood. Another friend, Rivky Senderovic, was the First Aid teacher there, and she recommended me as a substitute while she went on maternity leave. During my years in summer camp, I had earned my certification as both a lifeguard and a First Aid instructor, and I did a good job as a substitute. When Rivky came back, she switched to Biology and let me have the First Aid class.

This was the start of the 80s, when personal computers were just beginning to make their appearance. Rabbi Schenkolewsky, Bais Kaila's principal, was a real techie. He knew computers, loved to take them apart and put them back together again. Understanding the potential of the new technology, he set up a computer lab in the school. I was fascinated by computers and discovered that I had a natural flair for them.

People tell me that one of their favorite parts of my personality is my tenacity and stick-to-itiveness. My husband, brilliant as he is, can't read a manual. He gets impatient and starts riffling through the pages, hoping to find the answer to his question. Finally, he calls, "Shami! I'm stuck!" But I read manuals cover to cover. I understand them. Fortunately for me, there was an opening in the computer department, and I was given a job teaching keyboarding and a long-forgotten word-processing program called Electric Pencil.

At about this time, our financial support was running out and we needed to find other ways of making a living. Yossel was one of the best students in Beth Medrash Govoha, the world-renowned Lakewood Yeshivah. He could have taken the route that many of his friends chose and opened his own yeshivah. I'm sure he would have been very successful, because apart from a vast breadth of knowledge he also has plenty of personality and charisma. But he is a scholar and a writer at heart, and he wanted to study the subjects that interested him rather than focus on what his students might need. He was just finishing an important Hebrew volume called *Shufra Dishtara*, a treatise on the Talmudic laws of contracts, which he was hoping to have published, and he wanted to tackle other projects of this kind.

That was all very well, but how were we supposed to live? And how were we to pay for printing his book?

Confronting these needs, I came up with a solution. I would sell my diamond engagement ring and use the money to print my husband's book. If there was anything left, we would use it to buy a computer.

At first, Yossel wouldn't hear of it. But I assured him that I had no sentimental attachment to the ring, which was sitting in a safe because I was afraid to wear it. You see, I have a tendency to lose things. I know that after 120 years, people will speak about how I sold my ring to print my husband's book on the Talmud, but it was really no big deal. I was perfectly happy to do it. The book meant much more to me than the ring did. Okay, I like when people mention it. I just don't like when they make a bigger deal about it than it is.

Yossel is a brilliant Talmudic scholar, and I'm happy to say that his book has become famous. It is used today in high-level yeshivahs all over the world. I take much more pleasure in that knowledge than the ring could ever have given me.

As it turned out, we sold the ring just in time, because soon afterward the diamond market crashed. As it was, we had the money to publish the book, and with the money that remained, we invested in a computer.

After the crash, the financial support we'd been receiving from my father petered out. We were on our own. We decided to try and make a living by producing popular works on Jewish subjects for English-speaking readers. This would allow Yossel to continue learning in the yeshivah while earning a livelihood in the evenings.

Our first project was a translation of the classic *Menoras Hamaor*, a book of Midrash compiled in the fourteenth century in Spain. It would take three or four volumes to complete the work. If we could sell enough books, the venture might actually be profitable. I still had my job. We decided to go ahead and see what happened.

Yossel translated the first part, and I typed and formatted it. We inserted special codes for italics and other stylistic changes. Then we took the disks to a typesetter in Brooklyn. We saved some money by doing this, but by the time all the printing expenses were factored in we didn't make much of a profit. I also took in outside computer work, which brought in some additional income, but we were still short.

At that time, Yossel's study partner in yeshivah was Alexander Zissel Ellinson. His sister published an English-language magazine in Eretz Yisrael called *The Jewish Woman's Outlook*, and Ellinson, who is a very good salesman, was her distributor in the United States. During the 80s, Jewish schools and institutions would mail softcover books to potential donors as a fundraiser. If such "mailer" campaigns were run well, they could raise some serious money. Yossel suggested to Ellinson that they do a joint venture: He would translate excerpts from *Menoras Hamaor*, and Ellinson would find clients for them.

Ellinson made a deal for large-volume printings with Mifal Torah Vodaath. Those were the first books I sent over the modem to a graphics house in Manhattan — a great savings over the traditional route. Today, of course, it has become as easy as a click of the mouse, but back then there were many codes and protocols that had to be aligned before we could communicate by modem.

After several successful mailings, my husband and Ellinson decided to expand their horizons: they would form a corporation and seek additional clients. The name they chose for the company was C.I.S. One of their first clients was Bais Kaila, the local girls' high school. Ellinson made a deal with Rabbi Schenkolewsky to supply a volume of stories for use as a fundraising mailer. We commissioned the book. When it came in, however, the stories were not quite what we'd expected. We were dismayed. We had a commitment to fill, but no product to deliver.

Rabbi Schenkolewsky, the dean of Bais Kaila, was in a bind. He did not have a book for the mailing. I suggested to the rabbi that he ask my husband to write something for him. I knew that Yossel could do it, though he might not be that eager. I made the rabbi promise not to tell my husband that I was the one behind the scenes, pushing for Yossel to write a book for the mailing.

Rabbi Schenkolewsky called Yossel, who, of course, could not refuse. He locked himself in a room, where he wrote *The Promised Child* in five days.

Since he'd already begun to establish himself as a serious author of Talmudic scholarship, he decided to write this book under a pen name. We needed a pseudonym. For the first name he chose Avner, just because he liked it. He was groping around for a last name when I suggested that he use Gold, which happened to be the name of my friend's aunt. He shrugged. It didn't really matter, because we didn't think anything would come of it. We'd fulfill our obligation by giving Rabbi Schenkolewsky something for his mailing, and the book would be forgotten.

That's not exactly what happened. *The Promised Child* was a huge hit. People loved it and demanded sequels. But there was a problem. Yossel had written the fictional story without any thought to its historical context. He didn't know if he was in the fourteenth century or in the eighteenth. He hadn't even consulted a map. He'd known the main cities, and just made up the names of any smaller town the story required. Now he had to figure out exactly when the action took place. Without giving away the story, the only time that made sense was 1640. So that's when the stories are set.

Yossel went on to write another eleven books in all, which together became known as the *Ruach Ami* Series, by Avner Gold. More recently, he changed the name of the series to *The Strasbourg Saga*.

The eighth book in the series is *The Marrano Prince*. Yossel thinks it is his best book. It is set in Spain. Before writing it, Yossel studied Spain in great detail, using maps and travel books, but he'd never actually been there.

After *The Marrano Prince*, Yossel went on to other projects and didn't write another sequel for almost twenty years. In 2006, he was finally ready to continue the series. The ninth book, *The Long Road to Freedom*, was taking shape in his mind. It would be a direct continuation of *The Marrano Prince*, and the first part of the book would also be set in Spain.

Yossel wanted to see that country with his own eyes. Is it any surprise that this was the destination he'd chosen for our overseas trip?

As for me, Spain was all right, but my own sights were fixed on the Holy Land. I began planning my trip to Eretz Yisrael, that ancient source of wisdom and wonder. I wanted to daven at the graves of my ancestors and to ask for blessings from some of the great and holy people who live there.

Ten Days in Spain

Some time ago, Yossel taught himself Spanish. He actually speaks it quite well. He can communicate in Spanish, even if he sometimes has to add a smattering of sign language to make himself understood. He made the following offer to our son, nineteen-year-old Shulem: If he learned Spanish, he could accompany us to Spain.

Yossel gave him a book, and Shulem picked up a fair amount in the three weeks before our flight. We figured that Shulem would also be a great asset because he has an unusual ability to absorb maps and find his way around. He used to read road maps for entertainment when he was a little boy.

In August 2006, we flew to Madrid and rented a car. We were going to experience Spain without the benefit of tour guides or interpreters, just my husband with his decent Spanish, and my son with his limited Spanish and his map skills. We stayed in a hotel called Tryp Alondras, located within walking distance to the shul and the kosher restaurant.

On our first full day in Spain, my husband had arranged for a guide named Alex Benarroch to take us to Toledo. There are enormous billboard-size cutouts of black bulls on the roadsides in Spain, promoting the Spanish national pastime: bullfighting. Whenever we saw one, we called out, "*Toro*!" On reaching Toledo we passed a bullfighting arena near the shul, but it was closed.

The next day, we set out on our own. We drove to Cordoba. It was very hot. Very, very hot. We found a parking spot near the old walled city and went in search of the shul. We'd heard that it was in the center of the city and that there was a statue of the Rambam in front. This is technically true. But we had visualized something majestic. As it turned out, the shul was inside the walled old city, on a small back street only accessible by foot. It's a small building squeezed in between other buildings.

In the tiny square in front there does indeed stand a statue of the Rambam, but it is really, really small — about the size of a short person. Later, Yossel decided that a character in his book fleeing through Cordoba would go to that shul, contemplate that statue and think some deep thoughts.

Shulem suggested that we find out when the statue was placed there. It turns out that it was 1964. It would have been really funny if Yossel's character had seen the statue in 1684.

Well, maybe not so funny ...

The next day, we visited Seville, and on Friday we drove to Gibraltar, which is a British colony. It's a very interesting place. The road to Gibraltar passes through the airport. You drive across the runway when there are no planes landing or taking off. On Friday afternoon, we took a jeep ride up the Rock of Gibraltar and explored the caves.

There were families of Barbary apes, small monkeylike creatures, running loose across the top of the Rock. They don't really bother anyone, and people like to feed them. I was standing at the railing, eating a sandwich and looking out at Africa across the Straits of Gibraltar, when one of those apes charged at me.

Startled, I dropped my sandwich. The ape grabbed it and ran off. I guess I wasn't in any real danger, but the episode shook me up.

On Sunday, we drove to Malaga and Granada, and the following day we returned to Madrid. We still had a full day in Madrid, which we spent touring some of the city's famous sites. We went to the Plaza Mayor, where the last scene of *The Marrano Prince* takes place. And we visited the Prado, the world-famous museum of art, which was having a Picasso exhibition.

We bought tickets and had to wait outside. I sat down on the steps, suddenly feeling dizzy. Yossel and Shulem were deep in conversation with a fellow from Singapore who was waiting next to us. They were discussing the different languages spoken there. (Just in case you ever need to know, they're Chinese, English, Malay and Tamil.) They were deeply engrossed in their conversation and didn't notice that I was having trouble. I was suddenly overcome with fear, and for a few minutes, I thought I'd lose my balance and tumble down all those big stone steps. I felt totally off and instinctively tried to balance myself, though there was nothing I could use to brace myself. Fortunately, by the time I got their attention the dizziness had passed a little. I was able to go into the museum with them, still very shaky. The realization that I could fall at any time upset me, and I was subdued for the rest of the evening.

The next day, Yossel and Shulem saw me off at the airport on my way to Eretz Yisrael. Their flight home to New Jersey was due to take off a few hours later. On my return trip, I would have to come back through Spain and stay overnight. Yossel arranged with Alex Benarroch to pick me up at the airport, drive me to the hotel, and then return me to the airport the next day.

With a lump in my throat, I waved good-bye to my husband and son and was wheeled to the plane in a wheelchair. I was about to board a plane bound for Eretz Yisrael, and I was on my own.

My flight was uneventful, if a little tedious, and I was glad to set foot on solid ground again. My son, Berel, was there to pick me up. I saw the anxious look on his face, quickly covered up when he saw me in the wheelchair I had requested from the airline. He wheeled me out of the building into the glare of the broiling sun, and I was enveloped by intense, dry heat, so different from the humid summer weather back in New Jersey.

For a moment, an image flashed through my mind of myself as a young woman, a lifeguard in a sunlit girls' camp, slicing through the cool blue water in the Olympic-sized pool with an athlete's ease. With a sigh of chagrin, I put my hands on the wheelchair armrests and struggled to my feet, determined to make the most of this trip.

The Kalever wedding I'd come here to attend — the Kalaver Rebbe paid for half my ticket — was scheduled for the end of my stay. During the rest of my nineteen days in Eretz Yisrael, I was free to do as I pleased.

Precious Minutes

The country was experiencing a *chamsin*, an excruciating heat wave. I soon fell into a pattern of sleeping late in the mornings and venturing out only toward evening, when the day had begun to cool down. The first place Berel and I visited in Jerusalem was the big cemetery on Har Hamenuchos, where my father-in-law is buried.

My father-in-law, Aryeh Leib Reinman, had always had a fondness for me. After Yossel's mother passed away at the age of fifty, his six children all helped care for him. The married children took turns inviting him to spend Shabbos with them until his death at the age of eighty-four. He had liked me and he had loved Berel, his grandson. The two of us stood side-by-side at his grave for a long time, reciting *Tehillim* with deep concentration. The air seemed heavy with the intensity of our *tefillos*.

My husband and I have plots right next to my father-in-law's. We purchased them shortly after Yossel's father passed away.

The decision hadn't been easy. My father had expressed a desire for me to one day be buried beside my mother. Yossel wanted me next to him. What was I supposed to do?

Reluctant to hurt either my parents or my husband, I phoned Berel and asked him to consult with several rabbis in Eretz Yisrael. One rabbi stated that I should be buried next to my husband. Another suggested that I pick lots. But I would not be satisfied until I heard an authentic source in our holy Talmud to support this ruling.

Finally, Berel went to see Rabbi Chaim Kanievsky, one of the foremost Torah authorities in the world. Sure enough, Rabbi Kanievsky had the answer at his fingertips. "It says in *Maseches Semachos*: If her father wants her to be buried next to him, and her husband wants her to be buried next to him: If she has children, she should be buried next to her husband. If she doesn't, she should be buried next to her father."

I showed the response to my father, and he had nothing more to say. We bought the plots on Har Hamenuchos.

Our next stop was the grave of my great-uncle, the Pittsburgher Rebbe. I'd always felt close to the Rebbe growing up, and he could never thank me enough for what I'd done for his family.

I was just eighteen years old at the time, newly graduated from high school and working on Forty-Seventh Street in Manhattan. My cousin was to be married in Eretz Yisrael that week, and I casually asked his younger brother when he planned to leave for the wedding. He turned to me with a brave sadness in his eyes and said, "I'm not going. My parents can't afford the ticket."

I was upset. "What do you mean? You have to go!" Without a moment's hesitation, I declared, "Don't worry about the ticket. I'll pay for it. You can't miss your own brother's wedding!"

My cousin attended the wedding. Six months later, the *chassan* was dead of cancer.

My great-uncle never stopped thanking me for what I'd done. Every time he saw me, he would mention it again, much to my discomfort. After he died and his son succeeded him, the new Rebbe continued the same pattern, heaping thanks on me for that long-ago kindness each time we met. But I was repaid a thousand-fold, some years later.

I've always suffered from difficult pregnancies. Heartburn and nausea plagued my first two pregnancies, and a steady lower-back pain came along with my third. It wasn't until seven years after my third child, Berel, was born that I found myself expecting again.

I remember feeling so happy that day, in my fifth month, when I realized that I was well enough to dance a bit at a friend's son's wedding. Little did I know that the reason I felt so well was because the baby was no longer viable. We soon found out, however.

After delivering the lifeless child, I returned home in low spirits. When, a few months later, I learned I was expecting again, I was terrified. I'd heard about a kabbalistic stone that is worn around the neck to prevent miscarriages. I paid a deposit of one hundred dollars for the stone, which would be refunded in full when I returned it. I was not to take the stone off until my ninth month.

I tried to relax, though that proved nearly impossible. When my fifth month finally passed, I heaved a sigh of relief. Then, two weeks later, I realized that the stone was no longer around my neck. It had fallen off. The cramps began the next morning. It was all over so quickly that I had no time to mourn.

Beside myself, I phoned my great-uncle, the Pittsburgher Rebbe, in Ashdod. He heard me out and told me that as soon as I knew I was expecting again he would send me a certain *tefillah* to wear in an amulet around my neck. When I called him a few months later with the good news, he sent the *tefillah*, with instructions to wear it constantly until two weeks into my ninth month.

My son Shulem was born on March 29, 1987.

I went to my great-uncle's grave now, and cried, "You always liked me and cared about me. You gave me a special *tefillah* to wear around my neck when I didn't have a baby for almost ten years. You came through for me. Please, Fetter [Uncle], fight for me now. Daven to Hashem for me. You, who always had so much more concentration in *tefillah* than I will ever have, help me. Ask for a quick recovery for Shlomtza the daughter of Chanah Sarah."

I moistened the pages of the Siddur with my tears.

A few days later, we visited the ancient cemetery on the Mount of Olives, where Zaidiku, my great-grandfather, Bobby Ima's father, is buried.

Har Hazeisim, Mount of Olives, is located in the Arab section of Jerusalem. We hired ten men to join us and form a *minyan*. My son and I met them there and they led us down some stairs to a big building. Inside were my grandfather's grave and those of three of his sons. All of them had been great rabbis.

Away from the scorching sun, I stood in the dim stillness and poured out my heart to Zaidiku the way I'd done with my other relatives on Har Hamenuchos: "You are close to the Throne of Hashem now. Say a *tefillah* for me. Beg Hashem to help me. Because He is the only Healer."

After the relative cool inside the building, the sun seemed doubly punishing. I blinked in the fierce daylight and prepared to drag my feet back up the stairs. My heart should have felt lighter after all the prayers I'd poured out. But somehow, no matter how much I davened, there was always more waiting to come out.

Every second I spent in Eretz Yisrael was a precious gift that I could use to plead for my salvation, and I was determined to make the most of my time there. I'd gone to the deceased to plead for their intercession in Heaven. Now it was time to visit the living.

My son told me that he was taking me to meet the wife of a great Rosh Yeshivah in Jerusalem, Rabbi Nosson Tzvi Finkel, who headed the Mirrer Yeshivah with approximately 7,000 students, the largest in the world.

Rabbi Finkel also had Parkinson's disease.

Saving Lives

As long as I can remember, I was fascinated by the workings of the human body. Whenever I would visit or hear about a sick person, I needed to know everything about the illness: what caused it, how was it treated, what were the symptoms and so on. It was more than simple curiosity. I felt that if I had more knowledge I could help people.

When I was twelve years old, I registered for a lifeguarding course in the YWHA. That was where I met Ronnie. She was the instructor, and she was tough and demanding. She made me work like I'd never worked before, and I adored her. I discovered there was much more to lifeguarding than just swimming around in the pool. There was a lot of book learning as well: first aid, CPR and lifeguarding rules. As I said, I'd been a somewhat lackluster student in school, but to my surprise, I now excelled.

That lifeguarding course also marked the start of my lifelong fascination with all things medical. As an adult, I eventually became a certified EMT, an emergency medical technician, and I worked in summer camps as a nurse for a number of years. I also taught First Aid in Bais Kaila High School in Lakewood, the town where I live.

Even now, my thirst for medical information is unquenchable. I never tire of watching shows and films with medical themes, and I spend hours online researching medical questions. Ten years ago, a friend of ours discovered that his wife had a particular kind of breast cancer, and he asked me to help him. I did a lot of research and found a doctor in Dallas. They went to this doctor, and his wife is doing well today.

Believe it or not, I've actually saved a few people's lives.

My granddaughter Batsheva was once choking on a jawbreaker. Everyone panicked, but I performed an abdominal thrust on her. The jawbreaker popped right out and flew halfway across the room. On another occasion, at a family gathering, I heard one of my cousins screaming that her niece was turning blue; she was choking on a piece of pretzel. I immediately did some abdominal thrusts on her, but the sticky pretzel refused to be dislodged. I told my cousin to do a finger sweep while I continued the abdominal thrusts. It took three sweeps, but we got the pretzel out. The little girl was fine.

Mostly, I saved people's lives through my teaching. I always insisted that my students teach their families what they learned in First Aid class; and on more than one occasion, a mother has called me to thank me for helping her save her child from choking.

Thirty years ago, there was a family with a Tay-Sachs baby in Lakewood. Tay-Sachs is a genetic disorder that is mostly found among Ashkenazic Jews. Today, genetic screening can identify when a man and a woman are both carriers, a situation that places their children at very high risk, so that they can decide to seek other spouses. But this testing wasn't available then, and this young couple had two Tay-Sachs babies.

In Tay-Sachs, the babies develop until a certain point, and then they regress until they die, usually by the age of four. During this period, the babies are in constant crisis. I taught a mother with several Tay-Sachs children infant CPR, and she used it to save her babies many times. Eventually this couple moved to a different city, and we lost touch. Recently, she sent me an invitation to the *bar mitzvah* of one of her sons. On the invitation, she wrote, "I will never forget what you did for us. I'm forever grateful."

There was once a reunion in Lakewood for the alumnae of the high school and seminary in Gateshead, England. I was invited to deliver a brief talk on the subject of home safety. I suggested that all those attending bring a baby doll with them. There were fifty women in the room, most of whom I had never met. They'd all brought dolls with them, and I gave them a primer on rescue breathing, choking and CPR for infants. A few weeks later, I received a call.

"Are you Shami Reinman?"

"Yes."

"Are you the one who taught rescue breathing to the Gateshead alumnae?"

"Yes, I am."

"Well, Hashem should bless you! My son had a cold. The doctor gave me some medicine and told me that my baby would be fine. A little while later, I noticed that my baby wasn't breathing well. I was worried, but the doctor had reassured me that he was fine, so I just watched and waited. A few minutes later, my baby stopped breathing.

"Ordinarily, I'd have panicked and started screaming, which would not have been helpful. But I didn't panic. I remembered everything you taught us. I followed all the steps you showed us. I did rescue breathing over and over ... and my baby started breathing again! It turned out he had a bad virus, and he was hospitalized for five days. But now he's fine, *baruch Hashem.* You saved my baby's life. How can I ever thank you?"

What greater thanks can I ask for than such a call? The knowledge that people are alive and breathing and walking around because of something I did is simply incredible. It makes me happy.

But now, as I prepared to visit the great rabbi whose illness I shared, I was on the other end. I was the one desperately seeking advice to help keep me healthy, frantically collecting tips to help prolong my life.

My son and I took the short walk through the streets of Jerusalem to visit the world-renowned Rosh Yeshivah with Parkinson's disease.

Rabbi Nosson Tzvi Finkel, who recently passed away after a long life of accomplishment and years of suffering with Parkinson's, was a remarkable man. As the Rosh Yeshivah of the largest yeshivah in the world, he limited the amount of medication he took so that he could remain clear-minded. He ran the entire yeshivah, made plans for its expansion, took an interest in every student and managed, despite his illness, to deliver a *shiur* every day. Unable to stay in one place for long because of his spasming, he would speak using two microphones.

On the day I came to visit, I saw the Rosh Yeshivah walk into the house after delivering his daily *shiur*. He was so exhausted by the effort that he could barely speak. He whispered a blessing for my speedy recovery but was too weak for anything more.

I sat in the dining room and waited for his wife, Rebbetzin Finkel. The moment she walked into the room, I burst into tears. I didn't expect this to happen. It just did. She left the room quietly and returned a minute later with a box of tissues.

Mopping my face, I explained that I'd just been diagnosed with Parkinson's and was still in shock. I said I knew how important she and her illustrious husband were, and thanked her for taking time out of her busy day to see me.

Under the Rebbetzin's patient questioning, I poured out my story. I described my symptoms and told her about the medications I was taking. She insisted that I was taking too much medication and not taking it at the right times. She said I should take the medicine three times a day, during my waking hours, and not late at night when it would make no difference to my symptoms. And the drug Stalevo, she claimed, contains an ingredient that would prevent me from being clear-minded.

The Rebbetzin went on to tell me about the various things her husband had tried to alleviate his symptoms, such as a magnetic cap to wear on the head. She also mentioned a medicine that is taken intravenously, and a surgery called DBS, Deep Brain Stimulation, that can help with the symptoms of Parkinson's.

I stayed there an hour and a half, and with each passing minute, I became more depressed. This was a very serious condition. The long list of medications and cures didn't make me feel any better.

"There is someone I think you should meet," the Rebbetzin suddenly said. "His name is Rabbi Sofer. He's had Parkinson's for the past eleven years, and he's doing well. You should go see him."

And so, the next day I called the Sofer home. His wife, Chana, picked up the phone. I introduced myself and told her what I wanted.

"I'm about to leave for a water aerobics class. Why don't you join me?" she said.

I took a taxi and went to the class with her. It was an amazing experience. This method of exercising with weights in the water was perfect for me. You don't need as much balance for this kind of exercise. It would be a fine way to build up my muscle strength. I decided to try and find a class like this in Lakewood when I got home.

On our return to the house, I finally met Rabbi Sofer. My first glimpse of him was startling, to say the least.

He entered the house at a run, and stopped dead when he came to a chair that was blocking his way. As I watched in amazement, he jumped up and down a few times, like an engine building up steam, and then ran on to the head of the table.

Noting my surprise, he explained. "This helps me get where I want to go. For example, when I want to leave a room, I can run straight out the door ... if it's open. If it's closed, I basically freeze in place, and then jump up and down a few times to build up the momentum I need to open the door and leave the house." He smiled ruefully. "Sometimes, it doesn't work. Then my wife comes and opens it for me."

I watched him eat. He tilted his head all the way down to his plate and ate from the spoon.

"Why do you do that?" I asked.

He told me it was easier to bring his head down to the plate than the other way around. It took too much effort to lift the spoon to his mouth.

Afterward, he offered to show me some of the exercises he did. To my surprise, he went straight down onto the floor. I didn't expect a man his age to do that. He described his diet and his medications. He told me that he went swimming three times a week, with his son beside him to see that no one bumped into him.

He told me he'd had the flu and then pneumonia. He had been paralyzed from the neck down for four months, and had almost died. The doctors finally figured out that it was the antibiotics that were causing the paralysis. His wife urged me to make sure to get a flu shot, because Parkinson's patients should not get sick. They have a much harder time fighting any illness.

Mrs. Sofer, who'd never met me before that day, took the time to show me all the websites she and husband used to keep up with the latest medical information. She emailed all the addresses. I was in their home for many hours, and will never forget how nice and caring these people were to me.

My trip was drawing to a close. One day, my daughter-in-law Sora Rochel and I went to the Dead Sea, which is supposed to be extremely therapeutic for all sorts of ailments. But the simple trip ended very differently than I'd expected.

I was lying in the warm water, a little put off by its mineralish slickness but enjoying the incredible buoyancy that allowed me to float without any effort at all. Suddenly, my heart skipped a beat. Literally. My heart felt strange.

I'd read that expression in books and heard people use it in their speech, but actually experiencing it was a very different matter. I was worried, and I told Sora Rochel what I was experiencing. She insisted on calling Hatzolah. The ambulance arrived in due course and whisked me away to the hospital.

The attending doctors administered an EKG, and sent the results to my doctor in America. Thankfully, they were normal. Maybe it was anxiety.

At long last, I attended the Kalever wedding, around which my entire visit to Eretz Yisrael had been built. It was a beautiful affair, attended by at least a thousand people. I stayed close to my aunt's side the whole evening and asked her and the bride to keep me in their *tefillos*.

As I was preparing to leave the country, I called Dr. Adams, in the United States, and told him that I was very dizzy.

"You should have your ears checked," he said.

Is this guy listening to a word I say? I thought in disbelief. I was on five different medications, each of which had a warning on the label: "Caution: May cause dizziness." And he was advising me to check my middle ear?

In my heart of hearts I knew Dr. Adams was a top-notch physician. Nonetheless, I knew beyond a shadow of a doubt that I had made the right decision when I scheduled an appointment with Dr. Bressman. I needed a doctor who specialized in PD.

A Hug and a Kiss

August 30, 2006. My bags were packed and ready for my trip back to the States. I'd be spending one night in Spain before heading home. I left for the airport with mixed emotions. On the one hand, I was looking forward to seeing my husband and family, to sleeping in my own bed and getting back to my old routines. On the other hand, leaving Eretz Yisrael was always a painful experience. I always felt as if I were leaving a piece of myself behind. What's more, this time I knew that tremendous challenges awaited me at home. I faced the inevitable prospect of being sick and handicapped. Was I prepared to be that person? Not yet.

Berel brought me to Ben-Gurion Airport with plenty of time to spare. But there was a surprise waiting for us there.

"I'm sorry," a young woman wearing an airline uniform informed me. "You made a mistake. You're not due to leave until tomorrow."

Funny. Just like me to go to the airport on the wrong day. But it really wasn't my fault. My email ticket was in Spanish, so the mix-up was not so surprising.

Berel suggested that I'd been given a precious gift: a whole extra day to spend together in Eretz Yisrael. I agreed.

"Let's go to Bnei Brak," he said, "and visit everyone we didn't get a chance to see until now."

Rebbetzin Batsheva Kanievsky was the wife of Rabbi Chaim Kanievsky, one of the greatest rabbis of our generation. She was a great and extraordinary woman in her own right, and her passing not long ago was greeted with a major outpouring of grief from all segments of the Jewish world, especially women.

At the time of my visit, she'd become one of the holy landmarks of Bnei Brak. Every day, women and girls, as well as men, would line up to meet the warm-hearted Rebbetzin and receive her counsel and blessings. She seemed incapable of saying "no" to anyone who appealed to her in their hour of need. We'd been calling her home nearly every day during my stay, to see if I could get an appointment. We'd never managed to get through. But now we were going without an appointment.

When we arrived at the Kanievsky home, we found there was quite a line waiting to see the Rebbetzin. Two girls sat on the outside staircase leading to the Kanievsky apartment, controlling traffic.

"How do I get to see the Rebbetzin?" I asked one of them.

"Go upstairs," she said. "Ask which lady is last in line. You go after her." Berel armed himself with a *sefer* to study and decided to stay downstairs, while I went up to join the other women waiting in line.

It was a long wait. One by one, the other women asked me if I had an appointment. When I admitted that I didn't, they all went in ahead of me. Finally, I went back downstairs to consult with Berel.

He asked the girls what we should do.

"She can go in next," they decided.

But how could I do that? I didn't think the other women would take this well. When the door to the front room opened and I saw that it was empty, I went inside and sat down on a high-riser. Some of those waiting in line glared at me. I reassured them that I wasn't trying to get ahead of them. "I just can't sit on those plastic chairs anymore," I explained. They looked skeptical.

Suddenly, the door of the inner room opened and a sweet, smiling woman walked out. Rebbetzin Kanievsky herself! She came right up to me and asked, "Would you like to come to Maariv with me?"

Mesmerized, I gaped at her for a second, and then hastily collected myself. "*Lamah lo*?" I said. "Why not?"

I struggled to my feet.

She took my arm and led me to the stairs. The other women stared after us, mouths agape, as we passed by.

I was still too stunned to speak as we descended the steps. When Berel saw us, he quickly came over to the Rebbetzin. "Please daven for my mother to get well," he said. "She has Parkinson's disease."

We walked down the block to the shul, just the Rebbetzin and I, her warm arm holding mine tightly. We went inside and joined the service. Afterward, she asked me if I daven twice every day.

"No, just once," I answered.

"Daven twice daily," she advised, "and learn two laws of proper speech every day. May the answer to your *tefillos* come with your very next *tefillah*!"

As we walked out of the shul, a bearded man came over to her. She looked at me and said apologetically, "I hope you don't mind waiting. I have to speak with my son."

"Rebbetzin, it's really okay. I'll go now."

Her eyes opened wide. "What? You'll leave without a kiss and a hug?"

She hugged and kissed me, and I left with the warmest feeling I've ever had in my life.

Our next visit was to my grandmother's youngest brother, the Bukarester Rebbe. He was so happy to see us that we spent a full hour there. At this point I was still trying to keep my illness a secret and he had no idea I wasn't well. And yet, before we left, he told me earnestly, "Shlomtza, *ti mir a toiveh, zei gezint.* Shlomtza, do me a favor. Be well." If only he knew.

Then we went to the Nadvorna Rebbe, the son of Bobby Ima's oldest brother. In the month of Elul, the Nadvorna Rebbe, as did his father before him, does not speak during the daylight hours, and he does not speak with women. However, he made an exception for me. He had us come into his study to meet with him.

After hearing my story, the Rebbe said destiny had ordained that I go to the airport a day early, because I was not supposed to leave Eretz Yisrael without visiting him. He spoke to me for a while and gave me a beautiful blessing.

Berel took me to our next stop: a Kabbalist by the name of Rabbi Gamliel Rabinowitz. I sat alongside two other women in the waiting room. Someone was apparently very sick in their family, and they were constantly on the phone, making arrangements. I began to feel silly for being there altogether. I didn't feel too sick at the time, just a little dizzy and off-balance. What was I doing here?

But Parkinson's, as I'd read, is a relentless and debilitating disease. I might be feeling fairly functional right now, but things were going to get worse. What I had to do now was daven hard and collect as many blessings as I possibly could.

Rabbi Gamliel turned out to be a man who radiated happiness. After hearing why we were there, he handed us a jar of honey for the upcoming Rosh Hashanah holiday. And then he poured out something even sweeter: a heartfelt blessing for my speedy recovery.

My final day in Eretz Yisrael was drawing to a close. I'd crammed so much into the unexpected twenty-four hours I'd been granted. Armed with prayers, blessings, advice, honey, and the memory of the Rebbetzin's hug and kiss, I was ready to head for home.

A Book Is Born

It was a bittersweet homecoming. While I was thrilled to be back, the life I was facing included so many challenges: new symptoms, new doctors, new hopes and new disappointments. My dizziness wasn't getting any better.

Yossel shared my ups and downs as best he could, but none of this was easy for him. One day, he came up with an idea that was right up his alley, although I wasn't so sure if it was right up mine.

"Write a book," he said enthusiastically.

"A book?"

My husband is the writer in the family. Apart from computer and first aid handbooks, I'd never been one to immerse myself in the written word the way Yossel does. How did I know I could do it? And, even more, why should I bother?

"There's nothing as cathartic as writing down what you're experiencing," Yossel told me. "Put it all down, every stage of the way. What you're thinking. What you're feeling. You'll be surprised at how powerful a tool writing can be."

Looking back, I can understand why Yossel made that suggestion. He wanted me to have a goal toward which to work, something that would let me look back on my life and take pleasure in it. For another person in my position, the idea might have seemed ridiculous, but not for me. Books have been a big part of our life for many years.

While I'd never actually written a book before, I'd been involved in C.I.S. in the technical side of book production, learning to use the equipment and training the staff. I also evaluated and proofread manuscripts and did some basic editing. And I'd always enjoyed writing poems, although Yossel made fun of them. "That's not poetry. That's *grammen*!" *Grammen* are the cute, rhyming ditties that people compose for a party, poking gentle fun at the guests of honor and at themselves. Well, maybe it's not exactly poetry, but it does rhyme.

Although I had no experience with writing on this scale, I didn't reject the idea. Something about the project appealed to me, even as it frightened me.

"I wouldn't know where to start," I protested.

"Begin at the beginning. Start with your first symptoms, and take it from there. Give some background to put it all in context. And when you're done," Yossel said as the clincher, "I'll be glad to edit it for you. We'll get it published. The book will help not only you, but also other people suffering from Parkinson's and other illnesses."

Put that way, the idea began to seem more feasible. I began to actually feel excited about committing my life to paper, or rather, to computer memory. And if Yossel would give it a good polish when it was done, the book might actually end up as something that others could enjoy.

I looked at my husband. "I'll do it," I said.

Once I started, I became addicted. I wrote every chance I got. This was my tenacity kicking in, and that's a good way to describe my attitude toward putting my life down on paper.

Part of the book became an autobiography of sorts, where

I tried to introduce the person I'd been all my life. Much of the rest, my unfolding present-day life, appeared on the pages of my growing manuscript in diary form.

I found a certain catharsis in writing down the events and feelings that filled my days. Talking was becoming harder and harder for me, but I could still communicate my inner self to the world through the words that spilled from my computer keyboard onto the screen.

The hard part, I found, was putting it all down in logical order. I can be a very deep-thinking, orderly person, but when writing I'd find myself free-associating all over the place. One memory led to another; the timelines tended to crisscross and zigzag. I decided to write about things just as they came to me and let Yossel sort it out later. It became humorous. After every one of my falls or tests, I would make sure that someone wrote it down right away. I could be lying on the floor, pushing the emergency alert button and motioning to one of my kids, and I would say, "This was fall number thirty-six. Please make a note of it. I don't want to forget to put it into the book." My family took it more seriously than I did. I saw the funny side of it, and it helped me cope.

In trying to stay organized, I kept updating my manuscripts. I had piles of printouts with different versions and titles, and it was a great topic of discussion with my friends and family. I distributed chapters to all my visitors, and I had some very patient friends who helped revise my chapters over and over again. What came first? Did I get the shot first or the MRI? Everywhere one turned, there were boxes of earlier versions of my manuscript. I had drawers full of drugstore eyeglasses all over the house so that wherever I was I could read my manuscript. I always had at least some revisions to make. With the glasses, however, I couldn't see the letters properly, so I had my screen magnified many times. As a result, I had a hard time finding the cursor. I also bought an oversized keyboard.

This was getting out of hand. There were too many manuscripts, and I had a hard time remembering which versions were old and which were new. So we decided to save the files to

DropBox so that everyone could have access to them from anywhere in the world. Naturally, I had to give the password to all my friends. The problem was that we had many different devices, and one of my friends kept changing the passwords. That was when my troubleshooters came to the rescue. We were constantly busy debugging my computers and untangling the mess.

In Ilan High School, I was the computer instructor to all four grades. In the twelfth grade, we would produce camera-ready art for the senior graduation yearbook. As a teaching tool, I wrote some worksheets for Corel and Access that I distributed to the students. The worksheets worked wonders. For Corel, the students made basketballs, clowns and some original creations. For Access, which is a database program, I used a fantasy basketball league. The students were really enthusiastic. Even the weakest students were able to catch on and do surprisingly well.

My husband suggested that I turn the worksheets into books and publish them. We decided to call the series *Jump Right In*. The first book we attempted was *Jump Right In to CorelDraw*. We submitted it to my husband's literary agent, but the project went nowhere. So we decided to print the books ourselves. We stored them with Drop Stop, a shipping office in a local strip mall, and offered it for sale on our website. We didn't sell too many books, and ended up losing a few thousand dollars on the deal.

As it happened, a Polish company took note of the book and expressed interest in translating and publishing it for the Polish market. We sold the rights to them for eight hundred dollars. They translated and published the book and sent me a few complimentary copies. I have them in my den. They're conversation pieces.

So the only book I'd published so far was a CorelDraw workbook in Polish.

This would be my second. A very different kind of book, one with a medical theme. It would be the story of my personal struggle with Parkinson's disease.

I realized that this awful disease was slowly killing me, and I wanted to leave behind a legacy for my family and for anyone else who might be interested in what I'd been going through. Perhaps it would provide some encouragement and inspiration for other sufferers and their families.

Maybe, if I were really lucky, it would even be translated into Polish.

Making Changes

September was here, the start of the 2006-2007 school year. I'd been putting it off, but it was time to tell my principal that I was not well. In past years, I'd taught four classes, four days a week. Over time, my course load was reduced to ten periods a week. So I figured, why couldn't I come in just three days a week instead of four? That would make it easier for me to see my doctors and better for my health overall.

The principal shook her head when I made my request. "I'm sorry. I don't think we can work out a three-day schedule for you."

I took a deep breath, and told her the truth. "I've been having ... symptoms. I've seen many doctors, and they pretty much agree. Unfortunately, they think I have Parkinson's disease."

She looked shocked, and then deeply compassionate. "I'm so sorry, Shami," she said quietly. "I'll see what I can do."

They worked it out for me. That school year, I taught only three days a week.

Early in the school year, I also decided to come clean to my twelfth-graders: I told them that I sometimes didn't feel so well in the mornings. They were sympathetic, though a little puzzled.

There was something magical about teaching in that school. When I was in Ilan, I'd forget all about my various aches and pains. Especially when working with the seniors on their yearbook, which I did for many years; nothing could hurt me. Once, I felt a bit out of sorts but continued working. When I got home and took my temperature, it turned out I was running a fever of 104°, and I wasn't even aware of it.

Being the school's yearbook adviser, I often worked late. Yossel called me one night and asked how I was feeling. I told him I was fine. "You should get a night job," he joked.

That might be true, but I also knew that I was slower and sometimes felt a little dizzy. But I didn't let that stop me. I pushed through and got the job done.

That same autumn, I made another important change: I switched doctors.

Back in June I had scheduled an appointment with a specialist in PD for early October and the day finally arrived. Dr. Susan Bressman changed all my medications. Any change in regimen calls for some initial adjustments, and I found myself calling the office frequently to discuss dosages or side effects with the doctor. Each time, to my chagrin, I was put through to a Dr. Vicky Shenker, a fellow. This upset me. I didn't want my medicine adjusted without conferring with Dr. Bressman. I didn't realize that this was the way things worked with the busier physicians.

Dr. Bressman asked me if I would mind donating some DNA for a genetic-testing program being conducted for Ashkenazic Jews with Parkinson's disease. I liked the idea of helping in the search for a cure that would affect a large population of Ashkenazic Jews like me. So I went into another room and spit some mouthwash into a tube. It felt good, for once, to be able to give something back, to be part of a possible solution instead of just suffering with the problem.

This was a time of another important change in our lives, though not as important as finding the right doctor. After ten years of planning, we were finally ready to renovate our home.

We live in a bi-level on Steven Lane. Though it was not a very large house, I was very happy with it. Both my grandmother and my mother, however, had always wanted me to renovate the kitchen and install separate sinks for meat and dairy, but we were not ready to do it until the moment when we finally took the plunge. We added twelve feet across the back of the house and put in a new kitchen and new appliances.

My friend, Krassy Benedict, helped me choose the paint colors, the furniture and the living-room décor. We have many paintings, and Krassy decided how they should be framed and where they should be hung. When the job was done, we had a new formal dining room with a washing sink in the corner and a fourteen-foot table with fourteen chairs, and when we sat at the table on Shabbos, we felt that the room looked regal. It was a real pleasure.

I'd raised the question of leaving home during the renovations, but Yossel was sure we'd be able to handle staying in the house while the work was under way. The first night we stayed there, the bedroom was freezing. After all, it was late fall of 2006. The builders had taken down the outside wall. The next day, there was chalky dust all over the house, and we were choking.

That night, we moved into my son Chaim and my daughter-in-law Cindy's basement. During the good times, we used to go to them for Shabbos meal almost every week; they were always fun. I am very proud of Chaim. He is extremely smart, a great husband, a wonderful father and, of course, a devoted son. Whenever I need him, he is there. As for Cindy, she is a loyal and concerned daughter to me. She'd do anything for me. She talked to my doctors at length and researched every issue that arose. Now they were inviting us to live in their home until we could return to ours.

We stayed there for six wonderful months, from the end of November 2006 till May of 2007. We got to know our adorable grandchildren in a way that only living together can accomplish.

I became very close to them. Shalom Mordechai was eight at the time. Ari was seven, and Eli was five. Gitty was born about a week before we left. Chaim took Cindy to the hospital at six o'clock on a Friday morning, and we babysat the sleeping kids. When the kids woke up, we kept them home from school and drove them to the hospital to see Cindy and the new baby. Ezriel, the youngest, was born two years later.

I was so happy to be there for Chaim and Cindy when they needed me and to be a part of the beautiful experience of welcoming our new granddaughter when she came home from the hospital. In my opinion, that was well worth the price of being banished from our home for all that time. Not to mention the beautiful new kitchen waiting for me at the end of it!

During the time we were choosing and designing the new kitchen, I walked into the Advanced Wellness Center in Lakewood, which offers physical and occupational therapy. Standing right in front of me was someone who looked extremely familiar.

She stared as though she'd been thinking the exact same thing about me. "Aren't you the Mrs. Reinman who taught in the Talmud Torah thirty years ago?" she asked.

"Are you one of the twins I taught there?" I guessed that she was Arlene, but not wanting to make a mistake, I didn't say it.

She smiled. "I'm Arlene. I've had many teachers, but you I remember. I'm going to help you get better."

She gave me beads to thread onto a string. She also hung a fill-in puzzle on the wall so that I was forced to look up and stand straight to do it. I couldn't manage it. Then I played with Play-Doh to strengthen my arms. She was very professional and insisted that I rest between exercises.

"You go too fast," she said, "and you don't rest enough."

How could I rest? I wanted to get better. I was now taking occupational therapy, physical therapy and speech therapy. I was waking up at 3:30 or 4:30 every morning and trying to stay in bed until 7:30. I was desperate to make some improvement.

I mentioned to Arlene that I was about to put in a new kitchen. She smiled delightedly. "That's perfect! I'll help you. I'll come to your house and help you design your kitchen."

I smiled back at her, touched and grateful. You never know when you can make a difference in someone's life.

Arlene helped me lay out the kitchen. We also made one section of counter lower so that I could sit there with a regular chair and cut vegetables. It was a great convenience ... until the time came when I couldn't even do that.

I remember *that* day well, because it was Election Day (November 4, 2008). The Democrats were voted into power. I was optimistic that this could bring stem-cell research to America. They do stem-cell transplants in China now, and people are being helped. I saw an Internet story about a woman who had Parkinson's disease. She was very stiff and suffered from uncontrollable shaking. After she had a stem-cell transplant, much of the stiffness was gone, and she hardly shook at all anymore. She was a different person. She was able to function.

A ray of hope! I was determined to keep my eye on this one.

My husband is very close to Rabbi Aminadav Krispin, a Kabbalist who lived in Eretz Yisrael and made periodic trips to America. In January, 2007, Yossel and I asked Rabbi Krispin for his blessing. He listened carefully to what I had to say and then told me with great intensity that it was important for me to be *besimchah*, to live joyously. He suggested that I take walks on the beach and do other relaxing things.

He told me to say a chapter of *Tehillim* each day and ended our meeting with a heartfelt blessing for a speedy recovery.

He also made a remark that sent my mind spinning back into a painful part of my past.

"You are still grieving for your parents," he told me. "That is why your symptoms have come out in such a strong way. Your mother and father died within a few years of each other, and you were devastated emotionally." He gazed at me with compassion. "It is many years later now, but I don't think you've ever gotten over it."

I think he was right.

I Miss My Mother

Growing up, I was proud to be my mother's daughter. She was a very active woman, with a hand in every pie. Many of her days and nights and a great deal of her energy were spent helping the schools her kids attended and the community at large.

As a girl, I went to Bais Yaakov of Boro Park. My mother served as its chairlady and also as president of my brother's yeshivah. Many years later, during the week of *shivah* after her passing, Rabbi Ehrenreich, Bais Yaakov's longtime principal, told us that my mother had even picked out the bricks for the new building.

My mother was a people person. She knew everyone; and if she met someone she didn't know, she'd delve into their family history until she managed to find a mutual relative or acquaintance. Sometimes I'd squirm with embarrassment when she asked a perfect stranger where she lived, what her name was, what her mother's maiden name had been, in which shul her family davened, if she had any children and whom they had married. She didn't stop until she'd figured it all out.

Friday nights were a special time for me as a child. After my father and brother left for shul, I'd climb into my mother's bed, where we'd talk and laugh and fall asleep until the men came home.

After my marriage, my mother became one of my best friends. We spoke on the phone several times each day. If I didn't call her, I was sure to find a message on my machine: "Call your mother, you were only given one. Please call your mother, you have no other. Don't you miss your mother?"

My mother was a short, cute little lady. She was always dieting and always tasting everything. She loved to eat out and enjoyed treating us to a meal in a restaurant. One of her dieting ploys was removing the inside of the bagel before eating it.

I used to buy her gadgets designed to help her stick to her diet. Once it was a magnet for the fridge that said, "I eat like a bird, constantly." I think the best one she ever had was the talking gizmo. When anyone opened the refrigerator door, it would say, "Hey, are you eating again?" My mother broke that one into little pieces by the end of the first week.

My mother was a real character who always enjoyed a good prank. She owned a necklace of freshwater pearls interspersed with tiny gold nuggets. When my daughter, Devora, was twelve years old, my mother told her that the gold nuggets were the crowns from her back molars. At my son's engagement, Devora — by then married with children — wore the necklace. She was telling the necklace tale to my future daughter-in-law and showing her the actual pieces of tooth. My mother overheard her and burst into peals of laughter. Devora was shocked! What grandmother plays pranks? Well, I guess the apple doesn't fall far from the tree.

My mother never slept. Whenever you asked how her night had been, she would invariably say, "I didn't sleep a wink." She would sit at her computer; you could hear the tapping of the keys through the night. If I ever wanted a midnight snack, I had to tiptoe past the study in the hope that my mother would not hear me. She usually did.

I was the one who'd taught her how to use a computer, which she used to manage her mailing lists as president of the Ladies Auxiliary of the Rabbi Meir Baal Haness charitable fund. It wasn't easy to learn how to use a computer at her age, but she was a very determined woman.

There were three of us children: my older sister, my younger brother and me. Being the middle child, however, wasn't too bad. Mostly, I enjoyed it. On occasion, of course, I found myself fighting with either my sister or my brother.

There was one particular afternoon when I became extremely upset. I was overcome with self-pity. My sister, being the oldest, was the favorite. And my brother, being the youngest, was also the favorite! Where did that leave me?

I decided to run away from home.

Right from the start, I realized this was not going to be easy. I had no money, and I'd prepared no food. I decided to test the waters. I would hide under my bed and wait until they went looking for me.

I crawled under the bed and stayed there for what felt like a long, long time. It was getting dark out, almost suppertime.

"Hey!" I called indignantly. "No one even misses me! No one even notices that I'm gone!"

I slowly crept out from under the bed, went into the dining room and sat down in my seat. No one said a word.

It was two weeks before I admitted what I'd done. To this day, I still don't know if my mother had known about my escapade all along.

My mother was one of the neatest people I have ever known. I could never be as neat as she was, although I certainly tried. When we were growing up, my mother would sit at the Shabbos table like a queen while my sister and I took turns serving and clearing away the meal. We liked to surprise her by washing the dishes; she didn't buy a dishwasher until after I was married. She didn't need one.

At the table, my seat was next to my mother's. Every time I got up to serve, the chair got turned around so she could rest her arm on its back and be comfortable. I'd sit back down without turning the chair, and she would slowly inch her arm around my neck. Anytime I stepped out of line, I got a "tap" on my right shoulder, and a smile from my mother.

My mother talked to me and taught me and played with me. We loved board games. Scrabble was the family favorite when I was younger. If the letters were workable, it was a good game. Growing up in the Rubin household was loads of fun. There was always a game in progress. Up until her *petirah* my mother was in the thick of things and Scrabble remained the all-time favorite. Sometimes, my mother would get frustrated when she couldn't find a good word to put down, so we switched to Upwords. It was a much calmer game.

My mother taught me how to knit, crochet and embroider tapestries. We spent many warm hours together as she showed me how to do this stitch or that one.

I did not realize that my mother was aging. She was always sending my sister and me to help my grandmother — her mother — even though she herself was not a strong woman and could have used a hand as well. I remember the night my mother was walking down a steep stairway at a wedding with some difficulty. I looked at her, and she said to me, "You think at seventy I don't need any help?"

I ran to her, while the others continued assisting my grandmother. She rarely asked for help, and we never realized that she needed it. That was my mother. Sadly, she passed away before her mother did. We were not prepared for that. She wasn't the old one. Her turn had not yet come. At least that was what I thought.

I miss my mother. I could sure use her now. At the age of seventy, my mother was diagnosed with non-Hodgkin's lymphoma, a cancer of the blood. She was given two years to live.

I was stunned. How can this be? My great-grandmother, Malka, had lived deep into her eighties. Bobby Ima was pushing a hundred. I'd always thought my mother would follow in their footsteps.

Six weeks before she died, my third son, Berel, married Sora Rochel Kaufman, daughter of Rabbi Yechiel and Miriam Kaufman of the Sephardishe Shul in Boro Park. It gave my mother so much joy. I was happy to see the pleasure in her face. I was glad we'd been able to give her this gift.

The night before the wedding, I went to visit my mother in the hospital. As I approached the bed, she nodded her head at my father. I looked at my father, who took something out of his pocket and placed it in my hand. It was a pin and earrings set with opals and diamonds that my mother knew I liked. I used to borrow it whenever I came to New York and was wearing a certain suit.

It was a bittersweet moment. I clutched the jewelry tightly, trying not to think about what their presence in my hand meant tonight. I knew that my mother wanted me to have this while she was still living.

At Berel's wedding, my mother sat at the head table looking like a queen. Her face was sallow and she was very weak, but she sat there regally, a smile plastered on her face. The entire family formed a huge circle and held hands with the relatives seated at the head table. Everyone knew that my mother was very sick and that this would probably be her last wedding.

"Shami, do you think I'm going to get better?" my mother asked me one day.

"I hope so," I answered.

"You didn't say yes," she sighed.

Crossword puzzles were one of my mother's favorite hobbies. I would spend nearly fifty dollars each month on crossword books for her enjoyment. In the hospital, a few days before she died, I was sitting by her bed doing a puzzle. A nurse came in to take blood. We both heard my mother whisper something. I jumped up and asked her if she needed anything.

"Ask me the words you don't know," she whispered again.

"Did you just hear what I just heard?" the nurse asked me in disbelief.

"Yup, I heard it," I answered.

I asked my mother some of the words that stumped me. Sure enough, she gave me all the answers.

One afternoon, my friends Chaya Bodner and Leah Kreisworth came in from Lakewood to take me out to lunch and let me have a little break. My daughter Devora was there at the time, and she gave me a look of such terror that I decided not to go.

That was the day my mother died.

She died a few days before Tishah B'Av.

I was depressed for a long time. No one could touch me or make eye contact with me for two whole years. If my aunt, who was very close to my mother, would touch me or even look at me, I'd burst into tears. During the first, official year of mourning, one does not attend any sort of celebration. I learned, in person, why that is. It's because the loss is too great, and the one left behind is too sad. You cannot celebrate with a full heart at such a time. You just don't belong there.

Years later, I remember the family visiting my mother's grave on her *yahrzeit* on a hot day in July, 2004. I still missed her terribly. We went to the cemetery. My grandmother brought an umbrella to protect her from the sun. I decided to bring one, too. It really helped.

I could not stop thinking about my mother, and I lingered for a while after everyone left the graveside. The initial symptoms of my illness were just making an appearance and I was frightened.

"I know I'm not supposed to daven to a person who died," I said. "But I am allowed to ask Hashem to have mercy on me in your merit." I put my arm on the stone and I cried like I've never cried before. I said, "Mommy, what's happening to me? I'm sure you're crying for me and trying to help me. Maybe I was supposed to be even worse off. Maybe I should just make peace with this disease? What is going to happen to me? How far will this disease progress? What can I do to help myself? From whom do I need to ask forgiveness?"

I thought about my mother that entire night. Memories were popping into my head, piling up like leaves blown by the wind. When I look in the mirror, I see some of my mother's features in my face. I am the same height and we have the same build. I look down at my arm when I am wearing her wristwatch, and I see my mother's freckled arm. After she died, it took me two years just to be able to wear her watch.

Laughter and Song

My father, Rabbi Esriel Rubin, died five-and-a-half years after my mother. His father was the Dombrover Rebbe of Berlin, a scion of the Ropschitz dynasty as well as many other great Chassidic Rebbes. His mother, Chaya Bindiger, was a descendant of the illustrious Rav Elimelech of Lizhensk. My grandparents fled from Poland during the First World War and settled in Berlin, where they had a small shul in the Grenadierstrasse.

Being a Jew in Germany in the 1930s was not easy; being a Rebbe was even harder. On Kristalnacht, November 9, 1938, German soldiers broke into the shul to arrest my grandfather. My father's grandmother, who was very elderly, began screaming like a lunatic, pretending to be insane. Incredibly, the Germans left the shul without my grandfather and his family. A miracle from Heaven!

After the bitter night, it was clear the situation was only going to get worse. My father's family, his parents and three brothers, applied for visas to leave Germany, but they were only granted four out of the six they needed. My grandparents had to make a fast decision. Which children would they take with them, and which would be left behind?

After anguished deliberation, they chose their oldest and youngest sons, leaving my father, who was sixteen at the time, and his brother Mayer, only fourteen, with their grandmother until two additional visas could be obtained. My grandmother wept every day until her two sons finally joined them in America.

Somehow, the two precious visas were obtained. My father and Uncle Mayer were desperate to get on the last ship to leave Germany. To their deep disappointment and terror, they were turned away at the dock. But my father refused to give up. He kicked his brother and said, "Cry like you never cried before! Maybe they'll have pity on us."

Someone did. The two boys boarded the last boat to America. Another miracle from Heaven!

Although safe in America, the family lived in dire poverty. They had just enough to eat to keep them alive and no more. One time, they were at a *bar mitzvah* in New York, and my father was served a dish of sherbet. My father had never tasted sherbet before, and he just sat there staring at this incredible treat, savoring the thought of the new pleasure he was about to experience. Nearby, a boy asked his mother for another portion. Seeing that my father was not eating his portion, the mother snatched it away and gave it to her son. My father was stunned and devastated. He never got over it. Even when he eventually became wealthy, he often retold that story with remembered chagrin.

My father was reserved in public, but he was not that way at all with his family. He had the most wonderful sense of humor. He could tell the same joke over and over, and although we'd all heard it many times, we would laugh as if we had never heard it before.

I inherited my father's sense of humor. We were always telling jokes to one another, using a game we called the laughing meter. If he thought I'd made a terrific joke, he would give me 10 points on the laughing meter. If he thought it was terribly corny, he'd give me a score of 2. Usually my jokes and puns were pretty good, but he liked to give a lower number just to get a rise out of me. And when my father made a good joke, I would give him a 3 even though it was really an 8. We had a good time with that game.

Singing also played an important role in our family. Each year, on Rosh Hashanah and Yom Kippur, even after I married, I'd come with my family to stay at my parents' home so I could hear my father lead the Yamim Noraim *tefillos* at the Bluzhever shul at the end of their block. Although the acoustics in the shul were not very good, my father's sweet voice rang out loud and clear, and I would sing along with him under my breath. I loved the way my father led the prayers, and I wasn't the only one; people in the congregation always complimented him.

My father taught my sister and me how to sing. He would give us a single note, and we would have to harmonize along with it as he sang. If we hit a wrong note, he'd correct us by twisting his nose in a funny way. With time, we got better and better at it. My sister and I loved to sing the traditional *zemiros* with him at the Shabbos table.

On Sunday mornings, he would fix bull's-eye eggs for the kids so that my mother could sleep late. We enjoyed spending that time with him. When he came upstairs to say good-night to us, he made us laugh by squeezing us under the covers: He called them the *kvetchies*. Later, he played the same game with my children, and then my grandchildren. My son Berel now does it to his children, singing to them like my father used to sing. It's amazing how the little things, the small, precious traditions, are what keep my father most alive.

My father was a scholar. Whenever he had a free moment, he would go to sit in his usual corner on the couch, a *sefer* in his hands. He would sit there late into the night, until his eyes closed and he fell asleep.

When my father was about seventy, he spit up some blood in the bathroom sink. Frightened, he sought out a top surgeon in Manhattan whose name was Dr. Wu. The doctor had the utmost respect for my father. After his examination, Dr. Wu told him, "Rabbi, you have two choices: either shrink the tumor with chemo, or remove the tumor with surgery. There's a chance it might cost you your voice."

My father said, "I just want it out. I want the surgery."

Unfortunately, he did lose one vocal cord, and he could never speak again above a loud whisper. His beautiful voice was gone. But he did not become depressed. He remained the same sunny person he had always been. When he had to call someone, he would make a clicking sound with his tongue and smile. Yossel's aunt suggested that he continue to sing in his head, even if no one could hear it. A very good idea.

A few years after my mother died, my father remarried. He felt that if he didn't remarry before he was eighty, he never would. He was very happy with his new wife, and we are very close to her.

Nearly two years after they were married, there was a fire in the shul where my father davened on weekdays, and his *tefillin* were burned. He saw it as a bad omen, and he became very frightened.

Six weeks later, he was gone.

On a cold Shabbos in December, shortly before he passed away, we attended a cousin's *bar mitzvah*. My father and his wife were planning to go to Florida on Sunday, and they were looking forward to it very much. During the meal, my father looked very pale, and he fell asleep at the table. Waking with a start, he immediately made a joke of it, of course. He said that the speeches had been perfect. They'd provided him with a very good sleep.

But on *Motzaei Shabbos* he said he wasn't feeling so well. He took his temperature. It was 101°.

"Why don't you push off your trip to Florida until you're feeling better?" I asked. "Maybe you should see a doctor."

"No, Shami. I'm going for a whole month. I'll see a doctor there."

He got his way. He and his wife flew to Florida on Sunday. But later that first night, I received a frantic call from his wife.

"Your father doesn't answer when I speak to him!" she yelled into the phone.

A neighbor called the paramedics, and when they checked his temperature, it was a shocking 106°. They rushed him to the hospital.

We stayed up all night, waiting for a report. He was not doing well. We made plans to take turns going down there to be with our father. Unfortunately, I woke up with the flu the next morning, so it was my sister who flew to Florida to take care of him. I intended to follow, but my illness hung in there stubbornly. My brother, Naftula, went instead. I made arrangements to travel to Florida after Shabbos, but I was still coughing, so my sister flew back there again in my place.

The call came soon afterward.

"Shami, Totty has leukemia," my sister said, crying into the phone.

He was in critical condtion, and we knew that he could die at any time. My father had bought a plot in the cemetery next to his father, and if he died in Florida, it could take days until he was laid to rest, especially since it was almost New Year's Day, when the cemetery is closed. There is a strong tradition in Judaism that the soul experiences terrible anguish until the body it inhabited is buried, and we wanted to spare him the suffering. We chartered a medical transport plane with a doctor on board and flew my father back to New York, where he was admitted to Maimonides Hospital in Brooklyn.

I was there when he was admitted. I ran over to his bed and cried, "It's Shami. I'm here!"

He could barely lift his eyelids. I took his hand and said, "I love you, Totty." He squeezed my hand and struggled to open his eyes so he could see me. Then he smiled and closed them again.

There were a number of family members present in the hospital room, and we asked my father if he wanted them to sing the *zemiros* that he'd always sung on Shabbos. He nodded. His grandsons stood at his bedside and sang one song after another. My father's breathing was labored, but every time we asked if he wanted another song, he would nod again. They continued singing through the night.

Toward morning, I noticed that his breathing was not as labored. He had no more strength left to fight. We called everyone into the room. Slowly, as we davened beside his bed, my father stopped breathing. Totty was gone.

Since I became sick, I've often davened that he would intercede for me up above. Please, Totty! I know that you love me. Please beg Hashem to send me a *refuah sheleimah*, a speedy recovery. I'm so scared.

Prayers and Blessings

Unable to make peace with the Parkinson's diagnosis, we went from specialist to specialist trying to find the one who would have the magic formula. My first appointment with Doctor Lucien Coté was on January 14, 2007. His office was on the first floor of Columbia Presbyterian Hospital. He was short with frizzy white hair. He looked a little like the late world-renowned physicist Dr. Albert Einstein. Doctor Coté examined me and listened as I explained that I was dizzy, how my head felt as if it were asleep. When I stood still, he could see how my body moved forward and backward with no balance. He frowned and said that this was not the norm for a Parkinson's patient.

"I notice something else," he added. "Your eye movements aren't regular. When your eyes are closed, I can see them shaking behind your eyelids." He turned to Yossel. "I want you to watch out for this. Let me know if you see it happening, and if there's any change."

I told the doctor that I was having trouble using a knife when eating meat. He nodded his head.

"Parkinson's patients have trouble doing two motions at one time," he said. "For example, pressing down on the meat while sawing back and forth with the knife. If you concentrate and understand the movements that you need to make, you'll be able to do it."

I wanted to be optimistic, but reality was harsher than the doctor's encouraging predictions. The following month, I went back to school in the evening for parent-teacher conferences. Going upstairs, I stepped on a new carpet. Immediately, the room started spinning around me because the carpet was so plush. I swayed and became very dizzy. I got out of there as quickly as I could and met with my students' parents in my computer lab instead.

Almost as difficult as coping with my symptoms was the need to pretend that everything was fine. Everyone has to be an actress now and then. But ever since my symptoms started, I was forced to be an actress more and more often and in front of more and more people. It was discouraging. It was also draining. I constantly begged Hashem to give me the strength I needed to handle this test. And He did. Each time I felt my strength and hope ebbing away, something would happen to make things a little brighter. My encounter with my old friend and colleague, Mozelle Safdieh, was one of these things—a ray of sunshine coming through the dark clouds.

Mozelle and I are very close. In 1999 three fellow teachers, Mozelle, Frumie Feller and I, chaperoned the senior class on their graduation trip to Florida, and we've been friends ever since.

I hugged Mozelle, trying to pretend that I was the same old Shami she'd always known. She took one look at me and asked what was wrong.

I told her.

The next day, I received the following letter.

Monday, April 23, 2007

Dear Shami,

I heard your words, and I cried. I cried because you are my friend and you are in pain – physically and emotionally.

You are being challenged by Hashem on so many levels. We all get challenged, but when you are in the middle of one of your own, that knowledge doesn't make it any easier. No one wishes difficulties on others. We just hope to get through our own successfully.

I heard, and I smiled.

You are truly blessed. Your husband, children and children in-law are like the giant redwoods, majestic and magnificent in their love, caring and determined to help you navigate those very difficult waters.

I heard, and I cheered.

I cheered the love and strength of siblings doing everything in their power to add to a speedy recovery, and act as a second layer of support, but in no way second.

I cheered the extended family and friends (including yours truly) who will be praying and doing things to add to your merit, creating yet another layer of strength to help you reach the goal.

Ten years ago, I became a part of the staff of Ilan High School. I met you and some other very talented incredible women who touched my life with warmth and encouragement. We may be from totally different backgrounds, but we connected in a special way. Although we don't speak very often, and we find it difficult to grab a (private) moment for lunch, we share a friendship for which I am very grateful.

Over the years, Shami, you've been a great ear when I needed someone to listen, and you always have a no-nonsense way of giving advice that makes so much sense.

There is no trip that I care to take if you (and Frumie) aren't going as well. When you're there it makes it fun for me; those times are my best memories.

It's really amazing, Shami, and I don't know why, but I really feel you're going to beat this thing. You are not a quitter, and you can be tough. That is the fuel that is going to propel you.

I cry because it hurts me to know the battle you are facing. But in the same breath you give over so much positive energy that I feel you can only win.

Shami, you are my friend, your heart can read my heart. It is going to be some ride, and there are going to be times that you feel anything but strong. But you are going to keep on being the productive, accomplished and successful person that you are. Whether you teach twenty periods a week or eight periods a week; whether you do the yearbook next year or pass on it, it doesn't matter. Do what you can and don't push yourself to do what will exhaust you. Remember that real strength is doing what is good and right for you and those change constantly. (Taking a six-month break this year did wonders for me!)

Shami, you are really someone special. Thank you for sharing this with me. I know you know this, but I have to say it. If you need my strength (whatever that might be), you have it.

If you need my ear (anytime), you've got it. If you need my blood (I'm O+, universal donor – what else?), take whatever you need.

You can add me to the many fans that will be cheering every step you make toward that goal line!

I love you, Shami.

Mozelle

A Celebration of Life

My sister, Chayie, and I celebrate the same birthday, the day after Pesach. My mother did not have an easy time when she delivered my sister. She had a Cesarean section, which at that time was a serious surgery. Two years later, when she was expecting me, the doctor told her that a second Cesarean would probably be necessary. Since she was due around the same time, she decided that I should be born on the same date.

Now, many years later, I hardly had the heart to celebrate. My body had betrayed me and was slowly sapping the joy out of my life. But Chayie had other ideas. Right after Pesach 2007, she and her daughter Rivky came to Lakewood, to celebrate our birthday at my daughter Devora's house. People said that Rivky and I had similar personalities. We just clicked.

It was an anxious time for all of us. Rivky, my darling niece, was suffering from Hodgkin's disease. At just about that time, her doctor had found something in her lung, and she was due to be admitted for surgery at the end of the week. We were all worried about her. But we were determined to smile and make the most of the occasion.

I was surrounded by love that day. Cindy, my daughter-in-law, joined us for the birthday celebration. My son-in-law, Tzvi, called from Eretz Yisrael to wish me a happy birthday. Tzvi is the son of Rabbi Yochanan and Matty Follman. He is such a loving and devoted husband to my one and only daughter and such a wonderful son-in-law to me. He is caring, considerate, and always helpful. Actually, he is more like a son to me than a son-in-law. Whenever I need something, even if it's in the middle of the night, I know I can call on him and he'll be there to help and support me. And he is so much fun! When he comes into the house, with that big smile on his face, it's like a breath of fresh air. It meant a lot to me that he called from Eretz Yisrael on my birthday. Two of my students also called, as well as some friends. I was so choked up, I couldn't talk. It was an absolutely beautiful day. Afterward, Yossel and I drove my sister and niece back to Brooklyn. It was the least we could do.

It was April, a time when the whole world feels like dancing. As for me, it was getting harder and harder to simply get up from a couch. I felt as if I had the worst kind of charley horse. I did my best to ignore my cranky body and let my heart soar with the love I felt for my family and friends.

When we'd been together on my birthday, I had given Rivky my manuscript to read, as much as there was of it at that time. She finished it the night before she went into the hospital, and she texted, "I love you more than ever."

Rivky had the surgery. I davened and davened that she would have a speedy recovery. When she came out of surgery, she texted me often. It was easier to text than to talk.

A few days after her surgery, Rivky went into respiratory arrest. On May 3, fourteen days after the operation, she was given an additional name: she was now Alta Rivka. *Alta* means old. This was a desperate attempt to change her fate by changing her identity. She was placed in an induced coma in the intensive care unit.

Needing to do something to show how much I cared, I traveled to New York to visit my sister. My cousin Leah came with me. I felt this was something I just had to do. The previous Purim, my sister had traveled from Flatbush to Lakewood just to give me a hug and a kiss. How could I not go to Brooklyn now to be with my sister, at least for a few minutes?

I would have made the trip again and again, but my sister told me she'd rather have a sister who was well. If I insisted on coming that frequently, it would harm me both in the short run and in the long run.

One of my best friends, Rachel Novoseller, was marrying off a son in Montreal after Shavuos. I wanted to go by plane, but Yossel insisted that we travel by car. I had to admit, he had logic on his side. "Just in case we have to leave," he pointed out, "it's better to have a car. A plane does not always take off when you need it to. And it's not really so far."

So we drove to Montreal. Our son Chaim came along to share the driving with Yossel. In truth he was a lifesaver and drove most of the way both there and back. That's how we made the trip with one of the men at the wheel and me lying on the backseat of the car. At 12:30, just as the wedding was drawing to a close, Yossel received a call from my sister. Chayie said that Rivky was not doing well at all.

"What does that mean?" Yossel asked.

"*Baruch dayan ha'emes,*" Chayie said. Blessed is the True Judge.

Rivky had passed away.

We left immediately. My husband had been right. It was a good thing we hadn't flown. We would have missed the funeral. We drove through the night and arrived in Boro Park at 5:30 in the morning.

We went directly to the home of Estie Perla, my first cousin, and slept until nine. The funeral was scheduled for ten o'clock. The entourage stopped at Bais Yaakov of Boro Park Elementary School, where Rivky had taught. We saw all the older grades outside, walking with the casket.

The funeral service was held at the Novominsker shul.

Sholom, my brother-in-law, spoke beautifully, but it was painful to watch him talk about his Rivkala, only thirty-two years old when she was taken from us. Avrumi, her husband, spoke next and mentioned something that I hadn't even known about her. He said that Rivky had been a mentor for students in her school and often spoke to them on the phone in the evenings. Nevertheless, when he came home at night, she would immediately hang up and give him her full attention.

Rivky also used to visit my grandmother on Fridays, regular as clockwork. I never had to call and ask Rivky if she'd be there; she was. She also bathed my grandmother every Friday.

When visiting my grandmother in Boro Park, I would sometimes stop at Rivky's place until it was time to catch my bus. I slept there a few times, though she didn't really have room for me. She would put her boys to sleep on the couch so I could have their room.

Some time later, she moved to a bigger apartment. Rivky called and said, "Shami, I have an extra bedroom now. Please come to my house and sleep over. We'll have so much fun! Come see my apartment."

I never saw her apartment while she was alive. I saw it during the week that my sister, Rivky's mother, was sitting *shivah* for her. I'd never realized how big and beautiful it was.

Different Therapies

The following January, Yossel and I flew to Cleveland for the wedding of the child of a very close friend of mine. No one knew I wasn't feeling well, and I refused to use a wheelchair. Yossel had hurt his leg and was told to stay off it as long as possible. So he used a wheelchair at the airport while I struggled behind, carrying our suitcase and climbing the stairs.

Part of me was busy feeling sorry for myself, but another part couldn't help smiling. What a joke!

But it was becoming harder and harder to hold on to that smile. More than a year after my diagnosis, my symptoms were as distressing as ever. Apart from the aches, pains and limitations caused by my disease, I was also suffering from a debilitating dizziness. Wherever I went, I felt as if I were on the verge of losing my balance.

I was determined to commit to an exercise program to keep my muscles strong. We have a swimming pool in our backyard, so I resolved that whenever the weather was warm enough I would push myself to swim once or even twice a day, to try and keep my muscles from atrophying. At first, I couldn't get to the edge of the pool without a struggle. Gradually, with persistence and hard work, I got better at it. I felt good while in the pool, though the pains inevitably came back later.

One day, I was swimming with a friend. I was wearing a tee shirt over my swimsuit, and I wanted to pull off the shirt while still in the water. I turned onto my stomach and tried to pull off the sleeves, and I got stuck. I could not pull the shirt off, nor could I pull it back on.

My friend, knowing that I am a good swimmer and a former lifeguard, didn't realize I was in trouble. I was face down in the water, thinking, "I'm going to drown if I don't turn over."

Using my legs, I twisted my body again and again until I was finally able to turn over and maneuver myself back to the shallow water. I dragged off the shirt, my heart still pounding loudly in my ears. There is nothing like being helpless in the water to make you aware of your own vulnerability.

Eventually, I joined a gym, but when I participated in the water-aerobics class, I could only jog on my left leg because the exercise made the toes on my right foot spasm. Still, I enjoyed my time at the gym. I made lots of friends, and we became like family. Even after I could no longer go swimming, we all kept in touch.

Then an awful thing happened. The gym was sold and the new owners closed the pool. Most of the members switched to a different pool in Brick Town. I tried it once. It was a disaster. I slipped into the pool wearing my sponge noodle, ready for action.

"You can't come in here with a noodle!" someone yelled.

"Move over to the side or you'll get trampled!" called another.

That was it. This place was too crowded for me. I was just too fragile to use a public pool. Next, I tried a lap pool in a friend's house. But the pool had no stairs and the stainless-steel ledge was very slippery. So much for that idea. I missed the gym, where I'd been able to combine exercise with enjoyable companionships. Though I still felt eager for life, for connection, I was becoming increasingly isolated. I was losing the ability to participate in social functions.

During this time, my book was slowly coming along. I found that I enjoyed putting my life down on paper, or rather, on the computer. In a way, it was like a form of self-therapy. It made me feel better. And in the back of my mind I knew that when I finished it Yossel would whip it into shape for me. But writing, like everything else, was becoming an ordeal.

All my life, I'd always told myself, "Learn how to use your left hand. You never know when you might need it." Well, I needed it now. There were days when I had to type and write only with my left hand. I was getting better at it, but I still needed a lot of practice. I kept at it. I had no choice.

In the meantime, my condition was still a secret from most of my world. I was still trying my best to pretend I was functioning as usual. But it was becoming harder and harder to pretend.

The symptoms were persistent and excruciating. My toes hurt me almost all the time. Some of them felt as if they were broken; I couldn't straighten them out. When I tied my right shoe, my left leg shook, and when I tied my left shoe my right leg shook. My lower back ached and the middle of my back felt tight. I had to keep hitching my shoulders back to relieve the pain. When I got tired, I slurred my speech. I experienced shooting pains whenever I lifted anything or typed on the computer for too long.

Every day, I was getting slower. Every day, I worried about who would notice how long it took me to get out of a car or how I'd begun walking without swinging my arms.

Rolling chairs are called that because they tend to roll away from you when you try to sit on them. That's exactly what happened to me one day as I was helping my niece with her yearbook. I fell back and ended up on the floor. I couldn't stop laughing, but I needed help getting up. I knew that I'd lost my balance, but my niece just thought I was clumsy.

The next day, my side started aching, and it dawned on me that I might have broken a rib when I fell off the chair.

"If you really broke a rib," Yossel said, "you would be in terrible pain."

"I *am* in terrible pain," I said.

So we went for an X-ray. Sure enough, I'd fractured a rib in two places. I used this as an excuse when anyone stopped me and asked what was wrong with me.

"I knew you were walking funny," one neighbor commented. "Now I understand."

It worked for a while. I don't know why I wanted my illness kept a secret. I guess it was too scary to make it official. As long as I kept my condition to myself, it didn't seem as real.

It was also becoming harder and harder to speak. I found myself just looking at the words in the Siddur instead of uttering them. When I spoke to people, my speech was also becoming increasingly unclear. My darling granddaughters were such a help. They would look at me and instinctively know what I wanted to say, and they would often translate for my visitors. I finally heard what I sound like when I listened to a message I left on the phone for Yossel. I could not understand a single word.

After that, I'd have my friends listen to the message when they tried convincing me that my speech wasn't so bad. I saved the message for a while, but Yossel couldn't deal with it. He erased it.

Although I was struggling with my disease, I wanted to keep a semblance of normalcy in my home. I wanted the grandchildren to come by and spend time with me. Devora's older girls naturally started coming all the time and assisting me. Batsheva was eleven years old at the time, and Blimi was eight. They took care of me at home and accompanied me to weddings and parties that I wanted to attend. They were always there for whatever I needed, and practically lived in my house. Batsheva even helped me get into pajamas on numerous nights before I had a full-time aide. They laughed with me, and they cried with me. I was amazed that such young girls could have so much compassion and sensitivity.

Even in the midst of my suffering, I never stopped thanking Hashem for the blessing of my family. It was my love for them that kept me going.

Feeling Dizzy

The dizziness was getting worse. Was it the Parkinson's that was causing it? Or was it the medications I was taking? I decided to find out. I would wean myself off all my medicines and see what happened.

I discussed it with the doctor, and he agreed to the experiment. As the medication left my system, I became much stiffer. I tried to compensate by exercising in the pool as much as possible, but I had to be very careful. I fell over a few times and could not stand up from a lying-down position.

It was already mid-summer, but my head still felt as though it was full of sponges. I especially felt dizzy in crowds or inside a store. Pinny and Chaya Bodner, our friends for over thirty years, invited us for Shabbos. I could not sit long at the table. I kept getting dizzy.

Pinny had suffered from vertigo several months earlier, and he told me that he'd had gone to the Dizziness and Balance

Center in Lakewood. He suggested I see the same therapist, a woman named Robin. Maybe she could help me manage my dizziness. I wasted no time making an appointment. I was desperate to beat this thing.

Robin was helpful. She had me stand with my arms folded for thirty seconds and saw that I was moving and swaying a little more than the norm. Then she had me do the same thing with my eyes closed. I swayed much more, but I didn't lose my balance.

"You're doing fine," she said encouragingly. She placed a square sponge on the floor. "Now, do the same thing on this."

I was able to remain upright as long as my eyes were open. But the second she asked me to close my eyes, I fell right off the sponge. I could not maintain my balance.

Robin explained that because my brain has to work harder to keep me moving, sight was crucial for me. "I'd recommend that you keep a flashlight beside your bed, in case Lakewood ever has a power blackout," she said. "Without being able to see, you'll never make it out of the room."

I suggested that maybe it was my middle ear that was making me so dizzy. She had me lie on a table, where she looked into my ears.

"That's not the problem," she stated. "An ENG test is very uncomfortable, and you don't need it. There's nothing wrong with your middle ear."

As it turned out, she was wrong.

Robin asked me to describe the circumstances that brought on my dizziness.

"Every time I turn my head in any direction, I feel as if my head isn't going with me," I said. "I get this feeling in a car, in a store, or when there are many things to look at at the same time. Also when I have to walk through a crowd. I'm afraid someone will push me unintentionally, and I'll fall."

"In a crowd, you have to focus on something that is not moving. Look at a light fixture, for example."

She told me to turn my head to the side and focus on something on the wall. I tried it. There were various letters of the alphabet taped to the wall. I turned my head to the right and found an H. Looking to the left, I found an A. It worked! I didn't get dizzy!

"Let's do it again," Robin said. "Only, this time, I'm going to show you a card. I want you to tell me which card you see."

She whipped out one card, and then another and another in quick succession.

"It's the ace of diamonds," I rattled off. "I see the nine of spades. That's the jack of hearts." I looked at her in wonder. "I'm not dizzy when I concentrate on doing something else!"

"Now, walk backward and tell me which card I'm holding." Out came another card.

"I see the two of hearts. Now it's the six of spades. I'm going to fall."

"No, you're not going to fall. What card am I holding?"

"It's the four of clubs."

"See? You did it!"

She threw a few of the cards on the floor and told me to lean on my thigh when I picked them up. This would provide more balance.

I was excited about these new techniques. But would they be enough? I shared my fear with her. "I recently had a new grandchild, and I'm afraid to hold her."

"Okay," she said. "Let's play catch."

I caught the ball going forward. And then, even though I felt as if I were about to fall, I caught it walking backward.

"See? Your brain kicks in." Robin smiled at me. "If you can catch a ball, you can carry the baby."

I went home and held my granddaughter, Gitty, for a few precious minutes, tears running down my cheeks.

Detective Work

Bobby Ima was *niftar* 30 days after my darling niece Rivky. It was such a difficult period, but she must have made a big tumult in Heaven advocating for my recovery. A few weeks earlier, I finally (yea) got an appointment with Dr. Stanley Fahn at Columbia Presbyterian Hospital. Rabbi Shukey Berman had told us he is the best doctor in the field but it had been next to impossible to get in to him. He recommended that I take the autonomic neurological test. It was administered on July 12, 2007, in the same building as Dr. Fahn's office. As soon as I was done, I called Dr. Fahn's office to ask how to go about resuming my medication now that I'd taken the test.

The secretary put me on hold. When she came back, I asked her to please connect me to Dr. Collins, Dr. Fahn's fellow.

"I am in the building, Dr. Collins," I said when she came on the phone. "Can I please talk to you face-to-face instead of making decisions over the phone? I'm feeling worse since I stopped all my meds. I feel that it's important for me to be seen."

"All right," she said. "Come up to the third floor."

Dr. Collins took a videotape of me. She agreed that my right side was much weaker since she'd last seen me. She gave me a medication regimen, and we made an appointment for Dr. Fahn to see me again on August 6, when I'd be back on all my medications.

The medications took effect again. My balance improved, my handwriting was a little better, and my arm was swinging a little more easily. But I was still dizzy, slightly nauseous and out of sorts.

I called my daughter-in-law, Cindy, to discuss what to ask the doctor at my next appointment. She is so smart and organized, and I always rely on her to give me the best advice.

Cindy listened to me ramble for a while, and then she said, "Mommy, I'm listening to everything that you are saying, but it's not clear exactly what you want to ask. Let's be constructive. Let's make an organized list of everything you want to discuss. And make sure Totty takes notes, because you won't remember everything the doctor says."

She had me type out an organized list. It took us two hours to put it together. The list covered how I'd felt when I was off the meds and how I was feeling now that I was on them again. Then we wrote down all the questions I had for the doctor. Cindy was right. Making the list really helped me focus.

Dr. Fahn spent a lot of time with us on my next appointment. As soon as he saw the prepared list, he commented, "This is very good for your file. Let's go over it, step by step. I still do not have the results from the autonomic neurological test you took. I'll look into that. As far as your dizziness is concerned, let's try a patch behind your ear to see if that takes away the dizziness. It's like Dramamine."

So I put the patch on. The results were inconsistent. Some days I felt fine, but on other days the same old problem was back.

"Maybe the dizziness is coming from your inner ear. We should rule that out first." Dr. Fahn advised that I take an electronystagmography test, an ENG. "The test determines whether a balance or nerve disorder is the cause of dizziness or vertigo," he said.

Toby Bressler, my cousin's daughter, is the head nurse in the Columbia Presbyterian oncology department. She came down to meet me in the lobby after my appointment was over. I love Toby. She sparkles with joy, and she has a very big heart. We sat together for a while and laughed until tears rolled down our cheeks. If there's one person who can lift your spirits, it's Toby.

I met Dr. Shah, the ear, nose and throat specialist, on September 6. He looked into my ears. They were fine. Then he had a technician check my hearing. I sat in a glass-enclosed cubicle with headphones on my ears. The technician whispered words into his mike. I heard them all. My hearing was not the problem.

Dr. Shah then gave me a prescription for an ENG test to check if all was well with my middle ear. The ENG test was scheduled for September 17. Dr. Shah also gave me a prescription for an MRI of the brain, since I hadn't had one in almost two years. The MRI was scheduled for September 20, the day before Erev Yom Kippur. I could not sleep the entire night before.

The first part of the ENG test was not difficult. I sat down on a chair that was like a bed with the back propped up, and a technician put goggles on me. It felt like the kind you wear when you go snorkeling. There was a black strip in front of me, flashing red lights every now and then at different locations on the strip. I felt a little dizziness come on when I looked all the way to the right or left.

Right behind me, on the screen, was a camera showing my eyes. When I got dizzy, my eyes would shake on the screen. Both the doctor and Yossel were watching it. Here was proof, finally, that I had not been complaining for nothing. No doctor had understood me. Now here it was, live on the computer screen.

The next part of the test was the one that I'd been dreading.

"We'll just take some warm air and blow it into your left ear," the doctor said. "If you become dizzy or nauseous, just wait until it settles down, then look at the solid red light until the dizziness goes away."

After a few seconds of hot air blowing into my ear, the whole room started to turn around. I saw only black through the glasses, but I sure felt the spinning. Then the red light came on, and I stared at it until the dizziness subsided. The doctor then repeated the process in my right ear. My experience was more or less the same.

"And now," said the doctor, "for the cold air."

"What! I'm not finished? There's more?"

"The cold air I'm about to put into your left ear will cause the liquid in the middle ear to swirl around in the opposite direction. Let me know when you get dizzy."

The cold air blowing into my ear was not too bad; there was no return of the dizziness. The doctor kept it there for a while, just to make sure, but I did not get dizzy at all. Was this good news or bad?

Then the cold air was back, this time attacking my left ear. Dizzy! Very, very dizzy!

"So what does that mean?" I asked apprehensively.

"You probably have an infection in your left ear. Or some kind of inflammation. Dr. Shah will call you after he studies the results."

Here we go again.

Yossel was telling the family that I would take antibiotics to get rid of the dizziness. I, of course, was the skeptical one. I'd been suffering with this for over a year now. Couldn't it be related to my condition? Dr. Shah said this kind of dizziness is not what he usually sees with Parkinson's. So Yossel was convinced he was right.

On September 24, the Monday after Yom Kippur, I received a call from Dr. Shah, the ENT doctor. He told me, "I have the results from your ENG and your MRI. They show that you have a problem with a small blood vessel in your ear. This might be causing your dizziness and your balance issues. It may be an aneurism. I think you should see a neurosurgeon. That does not mean you need surgery, but he is the one you should see next."

I called Echo and spoke to Rabbi Konigsberg, who gave me the name of a doctor at Mount Sinai Hospital and one at Columbia Presbyterian.

"But I'm already going to Columbia Presbyterian for my Parkinson's," I said. "I've been seeing Dr. Fahn."

"Oh, then call him and ask his advice. He'll tell you what to do."

So I called Dr. Fahn's office. I hoped this wouldn't drag on.

Dr. Fahn thought a second MRI was in order. It was quite an experience. I was told to lie on a hard platform in a freezing room for an hour. They wrapped me in a sheet like a mummy and put a tape across my head to keep it from moving. A helmetlike guard was put in place to position the head. Then they placed a rolled-up pillow under my knees to make me more comfortable. This was a mistake. The pillow did not allow my feet to touch the table. After five minutes, I was already feeling uncomfortable. My thigh started tightening up.

"Three more minutes until the next part of the test," the technician sang out.

Three minutes is a long time when you're uncomfortable. I opened my eyes and realized that I was able to see a timer through a small window situated exactly at my eye level. I watched as the timer crawled to two minutes, and then one. I waited. The timer started again. They didn't stop the machine.

Oh, no, I thought in a panic. I have to clear my throat. I'm going to sneeze. Time seemed to stop. I would be locked in this machine forever. After five more excruciating minutes, the technician called, "Almost done."

They rolled me out and removed the pillow, ready for the contrast portion of the test.

"I don't have good veins," I told the nurse as she took my arm.

They never believe me until they start poking around.

"You weren't kidding, were you?" she said after the first failed attempt. She called in another nurse, who stuck me twice. Nurses can be very persistent. When they have no luck the first time, they don't give up. Instead, they maneuver the needle inside the arm, going deeper and using more force until they hit the vein. I was doing Lamaze breathing to get through the pain.

"I'm in!" she announced.

Back into the tunnel, this time for ten minutes. Then it was finally over. I was black-and-blue and swollen by the time I was allowed to go home. My arm pained me the rest of the night.

In general, I wasn't sleeping at nights anyway. Sometimes I'd doze off, but I didn't stay asleep. Any little noise, such as a doorknob turning or an alarm clock being set, and I'd be wide awake. Some nights, I simply didn't fall asleep at all. This night, with my arm throbbing with pain, there was basically no chance that I would fall asleep.

It wasn't much better the following night. I was so anxious awaiting Dr. Collins' call with the results of my second MRI that I had trouble getting even a few hours of decent sleep.

At long last, the doctor called to tell me that the MRI had been clear. "Isn't that good news?" she asked.

I didn't see it that way. I wanted answers. "If I failed the left middle-ear test," I said, "and the first MRI showed some vascular problem, then how could the second MRI show nothing?" I just didn't get it.

Seeing I was upset, Dr. Collins promised to speak to the radiologist again and get back to me later that week. After I contacted the office a few times, she finally called me back. She'd had another talk with the radiologist, who felt that the second MRI, which had focused on the relevant area of my brain, had showed that the vein was higher than originally thought. It was, therefore, not creating the inner-ear problem.

"You might have to learn how to live with it," Dr. Collins concluded soberly. "There are doctors who specialize in this area. They'll give you medication to help you."

All of life is a test. That's what I believe. Some tests call for making every possible effort to meet a challenge, to solve a problem, to overcome an obstacle. And other tests call for acceptance rather than perseverance, for embracing reality, for simply enduring.

But I wasn't about to give up the fight. Not by a long shot.

The search would go on.

Foiled Plans

Thanksgiving weekend 2007 was approaching. I was still trying to finalize my plans for the vacation break when Dr. Shah, my ENT doctor, advised me to take the results of my MRI to a neurosurgeon. I made an appointment at the neurosurgeon's office for November 16, arriving an hour and a half-early for a CAT scan he had requested.

Before I left home, I made sure to drink a lot of liquids so that my veins would be easier to find. When the nurse came in with the syringe in her hand, I told her, "I'm not an easy stick, Betty. My veins are hard to find."

Usually, when I warn the nurses they tell me not to worry, but Betty believed me. She pricked me two or three times without results. She tied a tourniquet very tightly around my arm, to bring my veins to the surface. She also put hot packs on my inner elbows, which supposedly helps the veins emerge. She slapped the arm a few times, looked it over and then switched to my other arm. The entire process was repeated.

"Ow!" I cried. "Are you in yet?"

"Not yet. I'll let you know." She pushed the needle further into my arm. "No, I'm not having any luck. I'll be right back. I'm going to get another nurse."

Doris came next. She tried and tried to find a vein. She thought she had one. Poke, push, prod. Nothing.

Finally, they decided to take me out of the CAT scan room so that it could be used for other people who were waiting. I sat down in a lab chair, and she resumed her search for a vein. She found a smaller vein in my hand and decided to go for it. Doris finally got the needle inserted. Then she called the doctor and asked him what to do next. It seems that the iodine for the CAT scan has to enter the bloodstream at a certain speed, through a big needle using a big vein. I had only a small vein and a small needle. Should they proceed?

The doctor told Doris to try it and see if I was able to tolerate the iodine in my veins when she pushed it in at a faster rate. All went well, and they proceeded with the scan.

Yossel was flying to Eretz Yisrael to attend the *bris* of our newest grandson, who would carry the name of his father, Aryeh Leib Reinman. Of course, I wanted to go along. I did not want to be left out of anything. Yossel promised me that it would always be my choice, but this time, I decided not to go. It would mean taking off too much time from school. Instead, I planned to visit Mindy Lankry, the daughter of one of my best friends, who was living at the time in Aventura, Florida, where her husband was the rabbi of the Sephardic shul.

At the last minute, I decided I wanted to go to Eretz Yisrael after all. I canceled my occupational therapy appointment, my physical therapy appointment, my appointment with Dr. Fahn and my flu shot. Then I called my principal and told her that I wanted to go to Eretz Yisrael and would have to miss a few days of school. She was happy for me and told me not to worry about it.

As the departure date drew near, however, I started sneezing and coughing, and my head ached. I went to the doctor, who diagnosed bronchitis. But how could that be? I had no congestion or wheezing.

"Let's try this," said the doctor. He handed me a weird tube. "Blow into this as hard as you can."

I blew into it three times, and each time, the marker read 270.

"What's normal?" I asked.

"About 500," said the doctor. "I'm not sure if your numbers are weak because of the bronchitis or the Parkinson's."

But I was sure. The coughing was not coming from my chest, but from my sinuses. It was the Parkinson's.

When I came home, I explained to Yossel that I didn't think it was such a good idea for me to go to Eretz Yisrael. I also told him that I'd had another of my premonitions. I'd known all along that somehow this trip to Eretz Yisrael was not going to happen for me.

He was looking forward to an overseas trip together with me, but he understood. "I'll cancel the reservation," he said.

I was happy to stay home alone, sleeping in my own bed and living on oatmeal and cold cereal. If I wanted company, I would call and ask for it. I needed to feel that I could take care of myself, even if it was a little harder than it used to be.

The day after Yossel left, he called me from Eretz Yisrael and told me that it was pouring. What's more, the room Berel had rented for him was a converted storage room, very cold and damp. That was just what I didn't need. I was getting happier by the minute.

On Wednesday, my daughter, Devora, offered to pick me up from work and take me for a stroll on the boardwalk, which is a few minutes from my school. We had only about five minutes at the boardwalk, but I enjoyed every one of them. Spending time with Devora is always a pleasure for me.

That night, Chaim and Cindy were going to a wedding and wanted me to babysit for a while. When I got there, I remembered that I had intended to go to a party, so they said they would come home early. A little later, Chaim called from the wedding to check on the kids.

"Are you having a good time?" I asked.

"We're having a great time," he said.

"Then stay as long as you want. I'm fine."

So there I was, typing this chapter on Chaim's new laptop, listening to a CD and babysitting my grandchildren. All things considered, I was content.

My Youngest Son

The day Shulem was born was one of the happiest of my life. It had been almost ten years since I'd given birth to my last child, Berel. From the start, we were extremely attached to our youngest son, and because we were older and freer to travel, we took him along wherever we went. Our other children kept commenting, "You never took us with you when you went away!"

When he was quite young, Shulem decided he wanted to see every state in the Union, and especially those that have famous bridges. Through the years, we traveled together to twenty-seven states.

We once went to Cincinnati, Ohio, to attend a cousin's wedding. On the way home, Shulem convinced us to take a detour south into Kentucky and Indiana before going home. That would allow him to add two more states to his list. We explained that doing that did not really mean he'd seen those states. This was the start of a debate between my husband and son that has never really ended. They would appeal to anyone who came to the house: "If your plane stops in England, but you didn't leave the airport, were you really in England?" Shulem insists that he could add England to his list, while Yossel maintains that he would not consider that he'd been there at all.

Shulem had a passion for puzzles. As a toddler, he would sit in his highchair and, after finishing a puzzle on the right side, would turn it over and do it all over again on the flip side. It was amazing to watch. He was a wonderful child who was very thirsty for knowledge. Shulem was interested in everything. I would go to the library with him and spend hours finding the right books.

We were once in the car on the way to New York when Shulem, who did not yet know how to read, piped up from the back seat. "Can we talk about the Civil War?"

Yossel's mouth fell open. "Sure, Shulem," he finally said.

"Who was in the South and who was in the North?" he asked.

How, I demanded, could he possibly know about this when he couldn't even read?

"Well," Shulem answered, "the encyclopedia shows that the South is red and the North is yellow. So I know!"

When he was four, Shulem loved playing a computer math game. The object of the game was to save someone, who was hidden in a submarine on the tenth level. On each level the submarine was guarded by a different type of fish that had to be avoided. The way to continue on to the next level was by answering certain math questions. The questions were more difficult with each level. The problems covered addition, subtraction, multiplication, division, decimals, fractions, rounding and progressions. In addition, the submarine was guarded by many sharks. Making one's way through a maze of sharks was not an easy task. If you were attacked by one, you either answered a new math question or you were out.

Shulem played the game without reading. Whenever I could, I sat next to him and read the questions out loud. Once, when I was in the kitchen cleaning chickens for supper, Shulem asked me to read a question for him so he could continue the game. I called back that I would come as soon as I could. A few minutes later, he came to the kitchen and handed me a napkin. I looked at it and saw the question he needed me to answer so that he could continue his game. Without knowing how to read, he had painstakingly copied down all the words.

I remember bringing home books about airplanes, puzzles, Lego, maps, populations, Civil War and the Guinness World Book of Records. At this point in his four-year-old life, I was interested in anything Shulem was interested in.

After that, Shulem began taking an interest in bridges, so I went to the library and checked out a book about the Brooklyn Bridge. I started reading it to him when I got home, but it was so technical that I put it down and offered to read a different book.

"No, don't stop! Keep reading!" he begged.

So I plowed my way through the rest of the book with my little boy drinking in every word.

A few years later, I took a job as a nurse in Camp Agudah Midwest. My older son, Chaim, was seeing a girl seriously at the time. Her name was Cindy Cohen, the daughter of Benzion and Bev Cohen of Baltimore. Chaim and Cindy became engaged on my second day in camp. I had to find a substitute nurse and take a car service to Chicago, and then a plane to Baltimore where the engagement party was to be held.

Ordinarily, such a trip to an unknown destination would have given me butterflies in my stomach. But I had Shulem with me.

My son, who was eight years old at that time, was very good at reading maps. Sometimes when I went in to check on him at night, I'd find him asleep with five maps underneath him. He knew the driving directions to most destinations in the United States.

Once, I urged him, "Shulem, tell Simcha how to get to Cleveland."

Tired of the game, he responded by providing exact directions to Newark Airport and told my nephew to take a plane.

Luckily, I had Shulem with me on that long trip from camp. Shulem knew the directions to any state in the United States.

With him there to guide me to Baltimore, I wasn't a bit nervous.

Now, as I battled my illness, Shulem was a young man in his twenties. I wondered if I would live to walk him down the aisle and dance at his wedding.

Friends, Students and Family

This condition of mine has been a big adjustment for everyone. While some of my friends call me often, I'm sorry to say that others avoid me. That hurts. I can understand that they feel less comfortable and are at a loss as to what to say to me, but it still hurts. On the other hand, I am getting closer to some of my neighbors, and some old friendships from the past have been revived. Some have become stronger than ever.

Chaya Bodner has been my closest friend for thirty-five years. After I got sick, she bought me a cuddly orange stuffed dog. When you pressed a button on the dog's paw, it sang a sweet, touching song:

Keep smiling, keep shining, knowing you can always count on me.

For sure, that's what friends are for.

For good times and bad times, I'll be there at your side forevermore. That's what friends are for.

Keep smiling, keep shining, knowing you can always count on me.

For sure, that's what friends are for.

For good times and bad times, I'll be there at your side forevermore. That's what friends are for!

I played the song for everyone who came to the house. The first five times I played it, I cried. It was exactly what I needed. I needed to know that my friend would be by my side no matter how sick I got, and no matter how much help I would eventually need.

Chaya, who works as a nurse in the nursery at Kimball Medical Center, has been by my side for as long as I can remember. When I was expecting Devora and I couldn't walk because of painful sciatica, she practically carried me into the chiropractor's office.

When I had my wisdom teeth pulled she stayed with me, fed me noodles and took care of me until I was able to take care of myself.

During one hospital stay, I woke up in the recovery room to see Chaya sitting there with a big smile and offering me ice chips.

I spent many sleepless nights worrying about my condition. I would find myself in my kitchen well after midnight, organizing my medical files on my laptop. One night, I was debating whether to stay on the computer or go to bed and finish the latest novel in a popular series. I'd started the series when I first learned I had PD. Losing myself in fantasy was a good distraction, and I really wanted to finish the book. Besides, everyone was talking about it, and I wanted to be involved. But this seven-hundred-page book was simply too heavy for me to hold.

Later that week, my friend Rachel and her daughter-in-law Dassa were visiting, and I mentioned the problem of the heavy book. Dassa was so concerned that she spent hours cutting the seven-hundred-page book into seven one-hundred-page ringed segments, each light enough for me to hold and read.

I couldn't get over it. I showed those ringed pages to everyone. This was one of the most thoughtful things that anyone had ever done for me.

As I said, some people have been avoiding me, but others are simply wonderful. Even on my darkest days, when I struggle with my symptoms and my fear, a part of me is glad that, because of my suffering, some of the people around me really shine. I bask in their light.

After she graduated, one of my students, Rochel Leah Abramson, became my assistant computer teacher in Bais Kaila. When she married, she moved to Eretz Yisrael, but we kept in touch. I'd also visit whenever I traveled to Eretz Yisrael. I received a letter from her right after she learned I was sick. Her letter really moved me.

> Dear Mrs. Reinman,
>
> I was shocked and devastated when I heard that you weren't well. My mind keeps conjuring up pictures of you with your ever-present smile and your never-ending spirit. I think of your love for life and adventure and your practical and creative way of approaching everything. I think of the energy and strength you invested into helping all of us, and your support and listening ear. I think of your hard-working nature and of your great strength in dealing with people. I think of you, and I am deeply pained by the knowledge that you are going through a difficult time.
>
> May Hashem give you the strength you need and send you a complete and speedy recovery.
>
> Thinking of you, Rochel Leah

Ilan, the school where I worked for many happy and productive years, holds an alumnae reunion every year. In 2005, I was totally flabbergasted when they decided to honor me. This was the first time they had ever had an honoree at the reunion.

I had not yet been diagnosed with Parkinson's at that point, but I was dizzy and a little out of sorts. My daughter found out about the reunion and told my daughter-in-law Cindy, my sister and my sisters-in-law. When the big night came, I was in for one of the biggest shocks of my life. The girls put on a slide presentation, similar to the one I used to produce for graduation every year. I'd seen them cutting out letters for a bulletin board and working on the computer and kept offering my help, but they always turned it down. I was too busy to check into it, so the whole thing went right over my head.

I have a feeling that they knew I was sick and wanted to show that they really loved and appreciated me. It made me feel loved but also sad. Bittersweet. Like so much else in life. But that night, it was the sweet part that dominated. My illness receded into the background as I felt the love surround me.

After the event, they handed me a scrapbook filled with notes and letters from my students, fellow teachers and family. I opened the scrapbook, and the first letter I saw was from my son Chaim:

> To my wonderful mother,
>
> Congratulations on this wonderful night. You really deserve it!
>
> Someone once said, "The reason Shami has good children (especially me) and children in-law is because she is a person who pursues peace. There is not a person in the world she doesn't get along with, or who doesn't get along with her."
>
> That is true, but I believe it goes far beyond that. You lead by your stellar example, teaching us what it means to be a respectful Jew and a respectful person. You are a role model to us, your children, as I am sure you are to each and every one of the students to whom you devote your entire existence. Your humor cannot be duplicated (corny jokes included). You have a way of making everyone feel important and special. You're the epitome of the person who is genuinely everyone's closest friend.

If we can only live up to ten percent of the example you set for us, Hashem will be proud.

May you always continue to make us laugh and to show us what it means to be a wonderful mother and a true friend.

Love always,
Your son, Chaim

I was very touched. Sometimes, sentiments such as these are not expressed to your face. It's easier to write them down, and I knew they came from the heart.

The letters from my students were also very heartwarming to me, especially because in many ways I considered them like my children. One student wrote:

Dear Mrs. Reinman,

It is very difficult to write on one paper how much you have done for Ilan and all the students, including myself. Year after year, I've witnessed you putting in your all into everything you do. Your persistence always pulled us through, and we always finished the work on time.

Through all the years, we already knew we always had you to fall back on whenever we needed a helping hand. Whenever we wanted an inspirational and fun weekend, we always knew whom to call, and you accepted us into your home with open arms.

When I heard this dinner was honoring you, I understood why they chose you. Out of all the teachers, you really deserve it. Your dedication to Ilan is awesome.

Thank you for all you have taught me, spiritually and academically.

Love, Laura Kassin

My granddaughter Blimi was eight years old at the time of the reunion. She and I are very close. When she comes into my house I always get a big hug, and she always runs without a second's hesitation whenever I ask her to do something for me.

Blimi found the scrapbook in my room and realized she hadn't written anything for me. She asked for a pen and paper. This is what she handed back to me:

Dear Bobby,

I lo♥e u so much!

You are the best grandmother anyone could have.

You are so nice to me. For example, you bring me to your school.

You let me come for Yom Tov and Shabbos sometimes.

Whenever I'm here, you always try to make me comfortable.

You know, Bobby, if not for you I would not be alive.

I l♥ve u so so much.

Your granddaughter,

Blimi Follman

Children, grandchildren, students are the greatest source of joy. I am so grateful for mine. So proud. And so grateful to them for loving me the way they do.

Another Dead End

My doctors say that if the room is not turning, then I'm not dizzy, so I coined a new name for my dizziness. I called it buzziness, and continued my efforts to discover the source. I came across the name of Dr. Robert LaRusso, a chiropractor. My cousin, Rivky Weiss, who suffers from vertigo, recommended him to me. At this point, I was ready to try anything.

Dr. LaRusso has offices in Manhattan and Staten Island, but he lives two blocks off Deal Road, which is right on my way to and from school. Unbelievably, he agreed to treat me in his home.

Now that I was no longer driving to school, I needed a ride to the chiropractor. I asked Crystal Green, an Ilan alumna, to take me there. When we pulled up in front of Dr. LaRusso's house, I thanked her and added, "Don't wait. This could take a while."

She smiled. "Not to worry."

As it turned out, she waited two hours.

Walking up the driveway to the house, I felt as dizzy as ever. I hoped Crystal wasn't watching me or noticing how badly I felt. I rang the bell.

A man of about forty answered the door. He was in his socks, which made sense as his house was carpeted in white. Dr. LaRusso took down my history and listened to the story of my dizziness.

"You're not dizzy," he stated. "You're suffering from a vestibular imbalance brought on by stress."

"But I don't really have stress in my life," I told him. I don't know what I was thinking.

"If you have Parkinson's," he said, "you have stress."

He had me lie face-down on the table, and the process began.

I never knew my arms had so many muscles. Dr. LaRusso tested every one. He poked and prodded and squeezed until pain was shooting at me from every direction. But that was only the beginning.

"Open your mouth," he said. He slipped plastic tubes on his fingers and placed his fingers at the side of my mouth. The result was so painful that I had to resort to Lamaze breathing to cope with it. He didn't miss a spot. Then he pressed the top of my mouth. More pain.

He went on to poke at other of my muscles, but between rounds he always came back to slip on those plastic fingers and put pressure on various places in my mouth. Each time, it hurt a little less than before.

Nearly two hours later, I got off the table. Dr. LaRusso had me walk around the table, and then bumped into me to test my balance. I was definitely less dizzy. Some dizziness came back later that night, but it was better than it had been before the treatment. Thoughtfully, he called me the next morning to see how I was doing.

Meanwhile, with Yossel still away in Eretz Yisrael, my sister Chayie and I decided to meet in Brooklyn and spend Sunday together.

"Let's go to Manhattan," I suggested.

My sister looked doubtful. "Shami, are you sure you're up to it?"

"Does it really matter? I have to push myself. I am not going to spend the rest of my life just sitting around. Let's go!"

Chayie caved in. She was beginning to get excited about the plan, too. "Do you want to call a car service, or go by train?"

"Let's take the train. I haven't been on one in years."

Sholom, my brother-in-law, dropped us off at the station. I clung to the railing, afraid to look down. We climbed the big staircase and reached the platform.

"Do you want to sit down until the train comes?" my sister asked.

Gratefully, I followed her to the nearest bench. If I'd known that the platform narrows there, I would never have attempted it. I felt as if I were about to fall right down onto the tracks.

Growing up, I lived on Fifty-Sixth Street and New Utrecht Avenue in the Boro Park section of Brooklyn. The train station was one block away, on Fifty-Fifth and New Utrecht. When I would see the train pull up at the Sixty-Second Street stop, I'd know it was time to leave my house. I'd run down the stairs, run up the block to Fifty-Fifth Street, run up two flights to the token booth, slip my token in the slot, run up the flight of stairs to the platform and make the train. That was my exercise for the day.

Now, here I was, some forty years later, barely able to make it up the stairs and petrified of falling off the platform. I held on to Chayie for dear life. But I was glad to be there. We were going to act like tourists.

We did a little window shopping but I found that to be too tiring. After a while we stopped into MOMA – the Museum of Modern Art. Some of the exhibits were beautiful and some seemed strange. But I — no we were having a blast. It was just a beautiful day.

I went home to Lakewood that night happy that I'd made the effort. There's nothing like a break in routine to put a smile on a person's face!

I told Yossel all about it when we spoke on the phone.

On the morning before he was due to fly back from Eretz Yisrael, he told me that he'd been davening for me with all his heart wherever he went. And then he was finally home. I cried when I saw him. It hadn't been easy being without him for two weeks.

We fell back into our daily routines. I went to see Dr. LaRusso again. He said I was much better. Two days later, I was as dizzy as if I'd never been to see him.

I had to face it. This was not going to be a simple thing to solve.

One morning, right after I got out of bed, I looked in the mirror and saw that my head was shaking slightly. I was afraid to tell Yossel, because he so wants me to get better. Whenever a new symptom appears, or an old one refuses to go away, I feel as if I'm letting him down all over again.

Numb, Numb, Numb

I was tired. Tired from lack of sleep, tired of my responsibilities and, most of all, tired of being ill. I wanted my old life back. I wanted my old bursting energy that I couldn't wait to burn up each day. I wanted to be able to function normally.

The pressures of teaching are constant, and I knew that the time was approaching when I could no longer handle the job. In the classroom, I was having a hard time double-clicking the mouse. The students could see that I was moving slowly. Getting in and out of my chair had become an ordeal. I had to lever myself by using my left leg and moving backward. My whole body felt stiff.

Meanwhile, I was struggling with my perception problem. It was very hard for me to watch the road while Yossel or someone else was driving; I constantly felt as if we were going to crash. I was always afraid that the driver — usually Yossel — would not brake in time and would hit the car in front of us. I kept telling him, "Brake! Brake!" This was making him crazy, and I have to admit that it was also becoming quite dangerous.

It was around this time that my creativity started kicking in along with my gradual acceptance of what was happening to me. Each loss motivated me to focus on how to find cute ways to come at it from another angle. I was determined to make our car rides enjoyable.

In my persistence, I found a way to download a Scrabble game onto my cell phone. That's when the fun began. We began playing Scrabble in the car. I would give Yossel the layout of the board and tell him if the word was in a column or a row and how far away it was from the edge of the board. Yossel would, from memory, play the game with me. Whenever we stopped at a red light, he would glance at the board to refresh his memory. He was always faster than I was, so he'd let me go first. We took turns putting down words, while Yossel drove us to wherever we were going.

This worked out very well. We were spending time together. I was not panicking every time he drew close to the car ahead of us, and my Scrabble game was certainly improving. One day, however, it became a problem.

"Yossel, where are we?" I asked, looking up from the game. "Why doesn't this road look familiar?"

We'd missed our exit.

I had a five o'clock appointment for a CT scan, again about my dizziness or rather my buzziness. We called the office and told them we were running late. Then we sat endlessly in front of a traffic light on Route One. Only four cars could get through before it changed again.

We came to the office an hour late.

"We're sorry," we were told. "The nurse waited for you, but she had to leave."

When I showed this little anecdote to a friend, she commented, "Where is your emotion? You have to put that in." She'd been following the progress of my book with interest, and I valued her input.

I thought about what she'd said and came to a realization that surprised me. Every time I get emotional about my sickness, Yossel always tells me, "Don't worry, you'll be fine." So I've learned to quash my feelings, way down beneath even my own radar, while I go on trying to deal with the practical hardships of the day.

Parkinson's does not come in full blast. Rather, it chips away, little by little, and ever so subtly, at every movement a person makes. If I complained last week about how hard it was for me to get up from a chair, I'd find that it's become a little harder this week. But I had already complained about it the week before. No one was interested in hearing the same complaint again and again. A person can complain once in a while and receive the sympathy they need. But no one is interested in someone who complains constantly.

I felt numb, numb, numb. How is a person supposed to deal with such a devastating disease?

Or was my numbness just another symptom of all the emotions I was suppressing?

Hard Days

My school took the girls on a trip to the Holocaust Museum, so I didn't have to teach. But it was not an easy day for me. I woke up at five in the morning and couldn't fall back asleep. Yossel offered to take me to the beach, but the weather didn't cooperate. We went to our favorite restaurant to eat lunch, but by the time we got there I was so dizzy — probably from not eating on time — that I couldn't enjoy the meal.

Yossel took me for a walk around the parking lot. That helped clear my head a bit. The minute we got home I went to sleep so that later that evening I'd be able to attend the *bar mitzvah* of my great-nephew, the grandson of my sister-in-law Feige Bulka.

When I woke up, it was time to get ready for the *bar mitzvah*.

"I'll be downstairs," Yossel told me. "I want to do some work on the computer until you're ready to go." He disappeared down the stairs.

Getting dressed had become a major hassle. In fact, it seemed to take forever. My shoulders would rise up and stiffen. I couldn't lift my leg to put my skirt on. I felt shaky, though it was only a few minutes after eight in the evening. I was supposed to take my medicine at eight; the few extra minutes should not have made such a difference. Why was I feeling so out of it?

I found it hard to pull down my shirt, and my sleeves were bunched up. I was aware of Yossel downstairs, probably beginning to feel impatient. He didn't realize I needed help. I couldn't get the lining of my skirt straight. I'd also been finding it impossible to tuck in my shirt. The right side of my shirt was always bunched up, because my right hand had become too weak to do it right.

I finally got my eye makeup on, though I didn't do such a great job. I came down the stairs.

Yossel called out from his study, "What's taking so long?"

I couldn't even begin to explain. Tears came into my eyes for the third time that day. I decided to visit the bathroom again. I always did this a few times before I had to go anywhere. By now, it was really getting late. I made a mental note to ask for help when I needed to get dressed for an appointment or an affair. I couldn't do this alone.

"If you want, I can go to the *bar mitzvah* with one of the kids," I said. "You can leave earlier. This is as fast as I can go, and it's probably going to get even slower."

When I finally walked into the *bar mitzvah*, I didn't even have the strength to go over to the mother or grandmother of the *bar mitzvah* boy to say, "*Mazel tov*." They must have thought I was a snob. I sat next to my sister-in-law, Perel, with Devora on my right. Beyond her were my sister-in-law Civia Cahan and then my daughter-in-law Cindy and my sister-in-law Miriam Reinman. Everything looked perfectly okay. To everyone but me.

Perel was talking to her daughters. If I ventured a word, she asked me to repeat it. "I've been having trouble hearing lately," she told me. Everyone around me was saying the same thing. It was so frustrating! I turned to Devora. She was talking to Civia, and I couldn't catch what she was saying. I asked her to lean back when she spoke. Then the loud music started.

I sat there trying to hold back the tears. No one was doing anything on purpose, but I found myself left out of every conversation.

I got the first ride home and got out of there.

Parties and crowded rooms had become a real challenge for me, but that didn't mean I couldn't throw myself into other things, if not with my former energy than with all the energy I possessed. Pesach was coming. The hype of the preparations was going on around me. I told my daughter that I wanted to be involved. We made the lists together, and I sat with my granddaughters, ready to peel vegetables.

I peeled one carrot. I was sweating. But I was determined to find ways to be a part of things.

The Seder was a real hurdle. Instead of helping my daughter and daughter-in-law serve the food in the kitchen, I had to let them giggle by themselves while I sat at the table listening to the men talk about topics that were not interesting to me. Whenever food was being served, I felt as if I were stuck between a rock and a hard place. I couldn't stand in the kitchen, and I couldn't stand it at the table.

Maybe, I thought, I should just sit somewhere on my own and read a book. I don't want anyone to feel burdened by me. They all do their best to make me feel happy and included, but all I can feel is loneliness.

At one of my therapy sessions at Tender Touch, Donna, the occupational therapist, had given me some recommendations for equipment to make my day-to-day living more manageable. It started with a stocking aid to enable me to put my socks on, a plastic footstool to make it easier to reach the floor, and a non-slip bath mat. She helped me order these items over the Internet. She also suggested that I have bars installed in the bathrooms and in the showers. She had me order a bedrail to help get out of bed, and a rollator, which is a walker with a seat.

Donna came down to the house, and we checked all the chairs in the house. She told me to put a towel in back of my head when I sit on the recliner. She also ordered ring splints for my fingers, to keep them from becoming trigger fingers.

With all of these new aids in place, I felt a little more comfortable getting around my own home. But then, unexpectedly, I was offered a chance to venture outside the house in a serious way. That January (2007), Devora offered to take me to Florida for four days.

Yossel thought it was crazy to do all that packing and traveling for a four-day vacation. But I didn't care. If Devora was willing to go with me, I'd take the four days.

Devora insisted we take a wheelchair along.

"If we have a wheelchair, we can come and go as we please," she insisted. "If we want to go to the mall, we'll just take the wheelchair and go. Ma, you know you can't walk around the mall for any great length of time. Right?"

Right, of course. But I was worried. "All my students are in Florida now. What if I meet them in a wheelchair?"

"Maybe it's better to start in Florida than at home."

We went to a medical supplies store near the Wal-Mart on Route 9. They have wheelchairs in the window display. As we pulled up, I saw a neighbor of mine, Tzippy Malavsky, in the parking lot. Oh great, I thought. Another person has to know I'm not well.

She came out of her car and said, "Hi, Shami. This is my store. How can I help you?"

Dragging my feet, I followed her into the store. This was so hard for me. Tzippy saw that I was antsy about the purchase and tried to soothe my nervousness. "You have such a good daughter who's willing to help you," she began.

That was all she had to say. I burst out crying. She handed me tissue after tissue, as I explained through the sobs, "I don't want to be a burden to my daughter. I don't *want* her to have to take care of me!"

After a while, I calmed down.

The store owner demonstrated all the different items that were available to help me. Then she commented, "By the way, I only take Medicare, so you probably can't buy anything here." She then told me where to go and gave me a list of the equipment I'd need. She was helping me even though I wasn't going to buy the equipment from her.

Well, I was so impressed that I bought the lightweight wheelchair. She had it delivered to my house.

As I'd feared would happen, word of my visit to Florida got around. Elyse and Frieda, two of my students, were coming to visit me in the hotel where we were staying. I looked at Devora with panic in my eyes. "How am I going to do this?"

My daughter had thought the whole thing through. "I'll bring you down to the lobby in the wheelchair, and then you'll sit on one of the chairs in the lobby. Don't worry, Ma, it's going to be fine."

We took the elevator down to the lobby and hid the wheelchair in a corner. Devora deposited me in a chair, where she propped me up with four pillows because it was low and much too deep. My students came. We talked and laughed. They didn't seem to notice anything. I didn't even have to repeat myself too many times.

When it was time to say good-bye, I smiled at them but did not walk them out. As soon as they were gone, Devora helped me back into my wheelchair and took me upstairs. We'd pulled it off.

Four days went by too quickly. We walked on the beach, and I must say I did pretty well. We talked a lot and laughed a lot. I went home more relaxed than when I'd left.

But every time I thought of what I'd had to go through simply to entertain a couple of students, I cringed. I didn't like having to hide my true situation from people. It hadn't been fun acting a part in order to fool those girls.

I felt false, as if I'd betrayed them. Just the way my own body had betrayed me.

I'd Rather Hide

Some days, I felt like hiding where no one could see me. On those days, the tears were right behind my eyelids, and just about any remark could trigger them. Sometimes I just needed a hug.

But most days, I was surprisingly upbeat. That was the way I'd always been before I got sick, and that was the way I tried to be now. No one is interested in being around a grouch for too long, no matter what the excuse. I tried to keep busy and find things to do.

It wasn't easy. I was so limited now. It was embarrassing to have to call a friend if I wanted to walk around the block or to shop at stores that provide a cart that I could drive around while making my purchases. I couldn't even cross the street on my own. I had to ask someone to call for me just to walk over to a neighbor's house, because I always felt as if I might fall off the curb if I walked by myself.

When I walked through a room, I looked as if I were drunk. Unless I hugged the wall or held onto something, there was a real danger that I'd bump into people. In a crowded place, I had to stay right where I was until the crowd thinned out and the room emptied before I could make an attempt to get through.

I learned this lesson the hard way. At one wedding, I waited for almost everyone to leave the row in which I was sitting. All I had to do was navigate around two girls who were in the way. Simple enough, right?

I started making my way toward the aisle. The first few steps were fine. Then I leaned over just a bit too much and lost my balance.

One by one, like dominoes, the chairs went back in slow motion, each one hitting the chair right behind it, which went on to hit the one behind it. Fortunately, I was able to regain my balance. It was still early on in my illness, so no one realized I was the culprit behind the collapsing chairs. I guess chairs are much lighter than they used to be.

My grandchildren hovered around me, trying to make me comfortable. They were sad for me. As time went on, they became more and more adept at easing my discomfort. My granddaughter Batsheva knew how to maneuver me in and out of a car. She knew how to hold on to me and shift me at just the right time. My granddaughters, Batsheva or Blimi, would come at night to help me get ready for bed. We would laugh when I got entangled in my clothes. And then we would cry. I am so blessed. I am showered with the love of my family and I shower them with my love in return. I feel that, despite my disability, I have a purpose in life. Even in my awful condition, I still make a difference.

I became the most competitive board game player, and the kids, youngest to oldest, loved it. I played Quirkle, Overturn, Uno, Racko and Rummikub with them. There was always a game in progress at my house, whether it was with family or the many visitors. And as it became more difficult for me to speak clearly enough to be understood, the games were the main form of our communication. They kept people involved, and they kept the mood light. We were having fun together. That is always good. But most of all, they were expressions of our love for each other.

If I wanted to go to a mall, I had to have a family member along or a close enough friend who was willing and capable of pushing me in a wheelchair. If I wanted to buy a dress, I needed assistance in slipping it on over my shoulders and off again. I then needed help paying for the dress at the cash register. I found it difficult to stand for too long.

By the end of the 2008 school year, I knew that I would not be going back to Ilan in the fall. I simply wasn't up to the job any more. The administration knew it, too. After all the wonderful years of non-stop action, teaching classes, developing relationships with my students, helping the seniors with their yearbook, chaperoning trips and relishing every moment of being part of the life of a thriving school, my teaching career was over.

The administration was very kind to me. I was offered a sabbatical with full pay, which helped ease my going. I was terribly sad about saying good-bye to Ilan. This had been a chapter in my life I would never forget. I'd forged bonds with some of my colleagues and students that, I hoped, would last a lifetime.

Every stage of life passes sooner or later. I just hadn't expected this one to end quite so soon.

That August, I spent some time in the Catskills, visiting my sister Chayie who is on the staff of Camp Chayil. Everyone I knew in Camp Bnos and Camp Chayil dropped in to my sister's bungalow to say hello to me. Each one came in with a different idea or gift for me. I was very moved.

When you're in a camp setting, everything moves fast, including new friendships. Goldie Schechter, whom I'd first met at a Bais Yaakov Convention, gave me a comedy CD to cheer me up, and then came over to watch the video I'd made for my sister's sixtieth birthday. Chayie's friend, the driver for Camp Chayil, drove me to meals and also took me to Camp Bnos to hear Rabbi Mattisyahu Salomon speak. Rabbi Salomon is the Mashgiach in Beth Medrash Govoha in Lakewood. When Rebbetzin Salomon saw me, she got up from her chair to greet me.

What an honor! I saw that it was hard for her to walk, too. The whole experience left me feeling pretty embarrassed.

On Friday, I was all packed up and waiting for my former student and friend, Rikki Epstein, the cook in Camp Shira, to pick me up from Camp Chayil. She was going to drive me to my cousin Esty Perla in Sackett Lake, where I would be staying for Shabbos. Two tenth-graders I'd taught in Ilan were in camp. I was really happy to see them.

"We heard that you're not coming back to Ilan next year," they said, watching me anxiously. It was clear that they were upset. I explained, without going into detail, that I was taking a year off for medical reasons.

This comforted them. I wasn't leaving the school just because I was tired of it. But it also made them more anxious. "Do you want us to daven for you?" they asked shyly.

"Yes. Please do." I gave them my full Hebrew name. "But I'd appreciate if you don't tell anyone else. I don't want to spread the word that I'm not feeling well."

The students solemnly assured me that they would keep my secret. They left with my name and the promise of their prayers.

I enjoyed that Shabbos with my family, though I tried to stay in bed as long as possible to avoid having to sit. The – to me – seemingly never-ending Friday night *seudah* had resulted in my staying at the table far too long. Did I mention that standing is really hard for me? Well, sitting isn't much easier.

At the meal, each of Esty's grandchildren stood and said a few words in my honor. They spoke simply. Nothing earth-shattering was said, but each one brought tears to my eyes. I cry so easily these days.

A New Diagnosis

On one of my visits to Dr. Fahn, he did something that surprised me. Instead of the usual Parkinson's, he marked down a new diagnosis on the insurance receipt. Possible MSA. When I showed it to Yossel, he was puzzled. As soon as I got home, I logged onto the Internet and looked it up.

> Multiple System Atrophy (MSA) is a rare neurodegenerative disease marked by a combination of symptoms affecting movement, blood pressure and other body functions; hence the label Multiple System Atrophy. Affected individuals may experience symptoms similar to those found in Parkinson's disease.
>
> Broken down, MSA stands for:
>
> Multiple - many
>
> System - brain structures that control different functions
>
> Atrophy - cell shrinkage or damage

MSA usually starts between the ages of 50-60 years, although it can affect people younger and older than this. The age of onset is usually 54.

Disease progression in MSA is quicker than in Parkinson's. Almost 80% of patients are disabled within 5 years of onset of the motor symptoms, and only 20% survive past 12 years. The mean survival is roughly 6 years. Rate of progression differs in every case and speed of decline may vary widely in individuals. It is rare for a patient to survive 10 years.

Patients usually have autonomic nervous system dysfunction first. When MSA begins with non-autonomic features, imbalance is the most common feature. This difficulty in maintaining balance may be due to either cerebella or Parkinsonian abnormalities. Some patients complain of stiffness, clumsiness or a change in handwriting at the onset of MSA.

MSA progresses over the course of several years to cause more widespread and severe symptoms. Orthostatic hypotension can cause fainting and falls. Loss of coordination, slowed movements and rigidity can interfere with activities of daily living.

Some patients with MSA have mild loss of cognitive abilities, with impairments in attention and speed of thinking. Complications include: progressive loss of ability to walk or care for self, difficulty performing daily activities, injuries from falls/fainting and side effects of medications.

Orthostatic hypotension (a large drop in blood pressure upon standing) is common and may cause dizziness, dimming of vision, head or neck pain, yawning, temporary confusion, slurred speech, and if the hypotension is severe, the patient may "faint" upon arising from a recumbent position.

In spite of low blood pressure while standing, it is common for MSA patients to have high blood pressure when lying down. A fall in blood pressure following meals or in hot weather or following infection is quite common.

The autonomic abnormalities are seldom the direct cause of death. A significant number of patients develop difficulty swallowing, which can lead to pneumonia.

Pneumonia is the most common cause of death, although irregularities in heartbeat or choking may be responsible for death in some patients. Breathing problems such as aspiration, high-pitched breathing sounds due to airway obstruction or cardiopulmonary arrest are common causes of death.

Currently there is no cure for MSA and no known means to slow progression of the disease. A number of drugs can be used to treat the various symptoms of MSA, although they become less effective as the disease progresses.

About 63% of subjects were unable to drive a car, giving this activity the highest difficulty score; 35% were unable to walk outside.

MSA is not hereditary, nor is it contagious. The mind of an MSA patient will be just as clear as any normal person's to the bitter end, even though one cannot express what is on his mind. Multiple System Atrophy is much rarer than its cousins Parkinson's or Alzheimer's. But unlike those two other brain diseases, Multiple System Atrophy does not have celebrities like Michael J. Fox and Ronald Reagan to publicize its cause. The end for a patient comes when the patient cannot swallow liquids or food and has to be fed by a tube. But most patients die before that due to complications from a fall.

MSA is a form of a slow but certain death sentence. Multiple System Atrophy is very rare. There is currently no cure.

The most promising treatment for Multiple System Atrophy lies in stem cell transfusions, but that is not going to happen in this country (U.S.A.). The Chinese neurologists are doing some interesting transfusions

> with embryonic stem cells derived from cord blood, but it is too early to tell their effectiveness or how long the benefits last. There are no guarantees in this unregulated industry. The Mexican doctors are also doing stem cell transfusions closer to home (U.S.A.). Any effective cure for MSA is still years away. In the meantime, the prognosis for MSA patients is not too bright. Current patients are not expected to survive long enough for a cure to materialize.

I read all of this with horror. Even worse was a first-person account by a man suffering from MSA.

> I would not wish MSA on my worst enemy! MSA wreaks havoc with all your plans and destroys your life. I wanted to travel, which would be hard to do from a wheelchair. Nothing below my waist is working and I can feel the numbness creeping its way upward above my waist. When it hits my heart, there is not much I can do since your heartbeat rate and blood pressure are regulated by your body's autonomous system which is out of whack in Multiple System Atrophy patients. My bank is calling me up questioning the checks I signed because my signature is not recognizable when compared to the signature card I signed twenty years ago. My speech is so slurred that I cannot pass a phone interview for a job.
>
> I still walk, but I am just one fall away from death. I have lost my wife and my family. Every morning I struggle out of bed wondering what faculties this disease has robbed me of which I had taken for granted before. Buttoning my shirt cuffs is a lost cause. Pulling on socks is a struggle.
>
> The MSA is affecting my digestive system. I choke more often when swallowing. I burp more often after I eat. My stomach is making more growling sounds after eating. I eat smaller meals more often. My digestive system is slowing down. I cough to clear my lungs every

> night when I hit the sack. My dizziness is getting more severe. I get tired more easily. The pain in my neck muscles is excruciating as it is harder for my neck to support my head.
>
> I am also suffering the effects of orthostatic hypotension (low blood pressure upon standing resulting in dizziness) every day. In a normal person the brain senses the lowered blood pressure upon the person getting out of bed (from a prone position to a sitting or standing position), and immediately the brain signals the heart to beat faster and harder to get the blood pressure up and to keep the brain from passing out. At the same time, the brain tells the blood muscles to constrict themselves to get more blood up to the brain. In my case, the message from the brain never gets to the heart and my blood pressure drops dangerously and dizziness follows. That is why the MSA patient has a tendency to fall due to dizziness when standing. I am not sure if this dizziness is caused by the progression of the disease or what. It is a sickening feeling, and I go through it every day.

I recognized myself in these postings, and I shuddered. If this was the kind of suffering in store for me, how would I ever endure it? How would I keep from going crazy? I have always had a low tolerance for pain. A trip to the dentist gave me nightmares. How would I be able to live with constant pain that was always getting worse and worse? How could I survive these final years of my life?

Back in 2007, I'd written a letter to "Ask the Expert" on the Parkinson's disease website. It read as follows:

> Dear Doctor,
>
> I am only fifty-seven, and I wake up often because of drooling. I have also been very dizzy. My head has pins and needles, and I can't look up or walk through a crowd. I weaned off the meds to see if that was the problem, but I was still dizzy. My doctor said I should take an autonomic neurological test. I was on Sinemet three times a day. I was

also on Mirapex, Azilect and COq10. I only felt a little better. Do you have any suggestions?

Here was the answer I got back:

See a movement specialist and have a PD scale called the UPDRS done in an off and then a super-on dose (2-3 tablets 25/100). See if there is a change. This may tell you or help you to determine if you have PD or a PD look-alike called MSA (or other).

It is important to get the diagnosis right before treatment.

Botox and anticholinergics as well as dopaminergics may be used for drooling.

Michael S. Okun, M.D.

There had been a hint that it might be MSA way back in 2007, but I hadn't taken it seriously. But I was taking it seriously now.

On our next visit to Dr. Fahn, we discussed his diagnosis. Was he sure it was MSA?

"No, I'm not," he said. "It presents as atypical Parkinsonism, and the rapidity of the progress of the disease and the kind of symptoms you are having strongly suggest that it is MSA. On the other hand, the Parkinson meds are having some effect, which suggests it may indeed be Parkinson's. It is impossible to know for sure without an autopsy, and hopefully we're a long way from that."

Hopefully. On our future visits, the doctor always waffled between Parkinson's and MSA, but in the end, he always leaned toward MSA. Deep in my heart, I believed it as well.

Memorable Occasions

The days marched on, some better and others posing a real trial. One day, when I was feeling especially low, I called my son Berel in Eretz Yisrael. I missed him terribly.

"Berel, you've been living in Eretz Yisrael since 2000. It's been nearly eight years already," I sobbed. "I don't know how much time I have left. Maybe you should think about coming home?" I cried and cried. I couldn't stop.

Berel didn't know what hit him. He couldn't sleep that night. His wife, Sora Rochel, called the next day.

"Ma, Berel is coming to America for five days. But he's coming on one condition: that you don't pressure him into leaving Eretz Yisrael."

Before I could say a word, she rushed on, as if she'd rehearsed this speech and wanted to get it out as fast as possible. "Berel is a respected rebbe in the Mirrer Yeshivah. He heads a *chaburah* of forty young married men. He doesn't come home for lunch or supper. He stays in yeshivah all day long and gets home at 11:00 p.m. He is also writing down all the Torah that he learns. You should be very proud of him."

I was. I was so proud of him. I was also a little ashamed of my outburst, but I was looking forward eagerly to seeing my son.

When Berel arrived for his all-too-brief visit, I apologized. I knew he was doing the right thing in staying where he was, but I couldn't help myself that day. I missed him too much.

Like all good things during this stage of my life, our time together was bittersweet. I enjoyed every minute of it but could never forget that he'd be leaving soon. The days rushed past until soon became now. It was time to say good-bye.

But this time, the good-byes were easier, because I knew I'd see Berel again soon. Pesach was coming.

Berel, his wife, and his six children, the youngest only two weeks old, flew in from Eretz Yisrael for the Yom Tov. I worked hard — harder than I was capable of — in order to get things ready on time. Devora had to clean her own house as well as help me with mine. We were finally able to start cooking on Erev Yom Tov.

After all the buildup, the Seder itself was a letdown. I sat at the table and watched the conversations go on around me. I could no longer hear what they were saying, since they were talking to each other and I was no longer included. These days, I didn't have the strength to join in unless I made an effort. I'd try to say something, but no one heard me. I'd try again, and this time everyone started shushing everyone else. "Sh! Mommy's trying to say something!" I felt stupid. Whatever I was going to say was no longer important. I'd look like a fool if I did and also if I didn't.

On Pesach, we relate the story of the Exodus from Egypt and the ten plagues. The next-to-last plague was darkness. Our sages explain that the darkness was like a dense fog around the Egyptians, and they were unable to move. This darkness was so heavy that one could physically feel it.

That's the way I felt. I was present in the room, but wrapped in a fog. I could follow a conversation, but no one heard me when I started talking. Everyone had to concentrate to understand what I was trying to say. And if there was any background noise or music, such as at a wedding, I might as well go home.

After my father had an operation on his vocal chords, he stopped going to weddings. "No one is going to hear me speak," he explained, "if the music is playing." Now I understood exactly how he felt.

I, on the other hand, still attended the occasional wedding. A memorable one was the day my niece, Rikki, married Yosef Baruch Reich, my friend Suri Jacobovitch's nephew. Yosef Baruch is now my husband's *chavrusa*, and they are both loving it immensely.

I rested most of the day of the wedding so that I'd be in the best shape possible that night. When we arrived at the hall, I paused at the door, eyeing the crowd with apprehension. Finally, I had my sisters-in-law form two lines, creating a set of walls for me to walk through so I wouldn't be shoved by the dancers and lose my balance.

Suri was delighted to see me. She and I had served together as head counselors in camp twenty-seven years earlier, and we'd been close friends ever since.

The celebration was in full swing when Suri, her daughters and other girls and women came over to the table where I was sitting and watching the dancers. To my astonishment, they made a big circle around me and started to dance.

Everyone around us stared and wondered.

"Who's that?" I heard someone whisper. "Is she a grandmother?"

I made them stop dancing. I saw the love that they had for me and felt bad about cutting the dance short. But I didn't want to be the center of attention.

The dance was brief, but the memory of that circle warmed me for a long time after the last of the music faded and the wedding was over.

The Hospital

The summer of 2008, I had my first really serious hospitalization. I was having spasms painful enough to stop me from breathing. This was something I'd never experienced before. My sister-in-law Shari offered to take me to a colon surgeon by the name of Dr. Glen Parker. Just getting there was an ordeal. Every time I stood up or moved my neck or back I would tighten up and spend the next few minutes trying to breathe through the pain. Devora held my back until, gasping and shuffling, I got into the car.

The spasms continued in the doctor's office. Dr. Parker waited patiently as I maneuvered myself onto the table. He examined me and then sent me to Monmouth Hospital to have my colon X-rayed.

After the X-rays were taken, my daughter said, "Ma, you look really sick, and I think you may have fever. I'm not taking you home like this." She called the doctor, and he told her to go straight to the emergency room.

They took my temperature every fifteen minutes. It was on the rise. Eventually, it would peak at 104°.

Chaim came that evening to relieve Devora and stayed all night and until the next afternoon. I was finally assigned a room. That's when the visitors started coming.

Wouldn't you know it? Tunie Missry, one of the founders and heads of Ilan High School, also volunteered for Bikur Cholim, an organization that visits the sick. She came to visit me, but the timing wasn't great. I had been given an enema, and I had to get into the shower.

My sister-in-law Feigie walked in next. She helped me put my two hospital gowns back on.

"My sleeve is stuck," I said, struggling. We laughed and laughed as I told her about my day. But it was nervous laughter, because we both knew that I was very sick.

It took a while, but my condition began to improve. Slowly but surely, my fever went down. On August 15, I was finally discharged. I went home swollen, black-and-blue, covered with bumps and bruises and coughing from all the fluids. I'd had an allergic reaction to Cipro.

After I got home, the doorbell rang. It was a nurse from the Visiting Nurses service. She'd come to take my temperature and blood pressure. I told her I could buy a blood-pressure kit in the drugstore. Remember, I used to be an EMT.

Blimp was the word that came to my mind when I looked down at my body. I'd gained ten pounds, mostly water and all of it in my legs, which looked like two tree trunks covered with red bruises and bumps, each as big as the top of a cupcake. There were bumps and lumps all over my arms, too.

I was finding it hard to breathe. I'd cough until I gagged. I felt as if I were drowning in my own fluids. Finally, the coughing subsided a little, but my throat began to hurt when I swallowed.

I was pale as a ghost and had bruise marks over my entire body, as if I'd fallen down six flights of stairs. An allergic reaction to Cipro takes a while to heal. It was forever before I looked like myself again.

I was weak as a fly. Devora rented a hospital bed for me,

thinking I'd be more comfortable. But I wasn't ready for that yet. Things were moving too fast.

She returned the bed.

My Students Shine

Throughout my years as a teacher, I didn't always know on which students I'd made an impression. And when I found out, it often surprised me. Another thing I'd discovered was that everyone shines at one time or another. You just have to be there at the right time to see it happen.

Rivky Kitay Ludzker was one of those students. I had had her in my class in Bais Kaila about eighteen years earlier. We'd had no contact since that time. Then one day, out of the blue, Rivky called.

"I've written a book," she told me. There was a touch of shyness in her voice, mingled with pride. "Can I send the manuscript to you?"

I figured she was probably hoping my husband would take a look at it.

She emailed the manuscript she'd just finished and asked if I would please read it. I had no strength at the time to read or write my own manuscript, let alone someone else's.

I hadn't been reading much since the dizzy spells had set in. Some days, my vision was disturbed as if I were seeing through a prism. On other days, the words were doubled or out of focus, and a letter or two were sometimes lighter at the beginning and end of each word. I wrote to Rivky, explaining that I wasn't feeling very well these days. I told her I was trying to work on my own book but finding it hard to do even that.

Rivky wrote back, saying that she had been sick, too! "I heard that you're also not well and that you're also writing a book. I'll read your manuscript while you read mine."

I was shocked to say the least. This was the last thing I'd expected. I dashed off another email, asking what was wrong with her. She wrote that she'd had a beauty mark that was dormant for years. Then it burst, causing a hemorrhage in her brain stem. She'd had to have brain surgery and was fighting a huge battle toward recovery. Therapy for her recovery was one of the reasons she was writing a book.

After that, there was no question of my refusing to read her manuscript. I settled down and began going through it, page by page, making corrections as I went along. And with each page, I realized more and more what an amazing person she is. It was a story of faith and strength during a terrible ordeal. I couldn't believe that this had been happening to one of my students, and I hadn't even been aware of it.

Many of Rivky's symptoms were similar to mine. But she, with Hashem's help, was getting better. I, on the other hand, did not expect to recover. All I could hope for was getting through to the end without more suffering than I could bear. Over and over, I reminded myself that Hashem loves me and wants only what is good for me. I clung to my *bitachon* in Hashem because He is my only lifeline.

Rivky came to visit me, but first, she sent me pictures of herself. As I said, I hadn't seen her since I'd been her First Aid teacher eighteen years before. She was anxious to see if I remembered her.

Of course, I did.

Rivky was living in Monsey, New York. My first impression of her when she came in was that she looked like a queen. She used her cane like a scepter. Her make-up had been put on to perfection. Her teeth were the whitest I had ever seen. As for me, I could barely brush my teeth. How is she able to do that? I wondered. I could never look so put together.

I wondered if it was the diet and health food that was helping her get better. Rivky offered to come with me when I went to my nutritionist. She was eager to share her strength and advice.

We spoke to each other often, and that trip in her van was only the first of many visits. She helped me so much. She made me nutritious soups and offered me healthy recipes. Rivky and I emailed each other almost daily.

During this period, Rebbetzin Hoberman, a former principal of Bais Kaila, passed away in November 2008. Although she was the Hebrew principal and I taught First Aid and Computers in the general studies department, we had become friends. During her illness, I'd gone to visit her. I'd felt very close to Rebbetzin Hoberman, and I knew that her loss would be a great loss to me, to Lakewood and to the rest of the world.

Thirty days after Rebbetzin Hoberman's passing, a *sheloshim,* commemorative gathering, was held in her honor. Despite my fear of crowds, I attended. As I'd expected, the room was packed. Many of her students came to pay their respects.

Quite a few members of the family came over to me. I could tell, by the way they squeezed my hand or hugged me, which ones knew I wasn't well and which didn't. Many of my former students came over, too, just to say hello.

It was the first time I was at a big gathering where everyone knew me. I was very nervous. I tried to make myself inconspicuous, but it was a lost cause.

The speeches began. And so did my movements. First, my shoulder started going up and down, and then my neck got involved. My right arm joined in and my toes did a dance. The doctors call these involuntary movements dyskinesia. They happened every time I used my right arm. Every word I typed was accompanied by movements involving my neck, shoulders, arms and toes.

I sat during those speeches struggling with the dyskinesia and losing the battle. The more I tried to relax, the worse it got.

I'd chosen a seat in the third row. That was a big mistake. The second-to-last row would have been better. When I had to go out in public, I usually came late so that fewer people would see me and left early so that I wouldn't have to cope with the crowds and risk being trampled.

I don't know how many people saw me that night, but I do know that if I'd wanted to advertise that I was sick, I'd done exactly the right thing.

Faiga Cukier Gross, a former student from Bais Kaila, saw me at that gathering. At the time, I was leaning on another former student, Rivka Leah Jacobovitch Schechter, for support. Faiga called Rivka Leah that same night and asked, "What is going on with Mrs. Reinman?"

Rivka Leah told her that I was having muscle problems.

From that day on, Faiga was there for me. She called me almost every day.

"Can I pick you up and take you to Mrs. Schwartzman for a massage this morning? I'll pick you up at 9:30. Does that work for you?"

"Do you need any almond flour?"

"Have you ever tried Oriental therapies?"

"Do you have this cookie recipe? I'll bring some over for you to taste."

Faiga and Rivka joined forces and created a recipe book for me containing all their healthy recipes. They took me off milk, white flour and sugar. Rivky made me soups and Faiga sent me cookies. I was growing fatter.

Over the years, different students had kept in touch through emails or text messages. Some took me out for diet ice cream, and some just came to visit. And then there were those who said they would come or call but either didn't have the time or found that they couldn't cope with it.

I didn't hold that against them. Not everybody can handle seeing a once-healthy body slowly deteriorating. Even I wasn't handling it so well, and it was happening to me!

But, all in all, the students from my teaching years had been, and continued to be, a light in my life, a warm, living connection between the person I'd been and the one I was today. Their love and concern were bright spots in my day. And I'm sure they knew, or I hoped they knew, that I felt exactly the same way about each and every one of them.

A Roller-Coaster Ride

My feet had developed bunions and were hurting me very much. I made an appointment with Dr. Hubbard, an orthopedist, for 10:30 a.m. on March 11 to determine if I needed surgery. Later that day, I had an appointment with Dr. Fahn, my PD doctor. With so much on the schedule, I set the alarm for 6:00 but was so afraid that I wouldn't get up on time that I couldn't fall asleep. I drifted off at about 1:00 a.m. and woke up suddenly two hours later. Immediately, I knew that going back to sleep was not an option. I was too wired-up to sleep. So I went down to my computer to prepare my questions for the doctors.

"I need you to keep a daily log," Dr. Fahn had explained. So, each day, I used my phone to keep a log of how I was feeling. Then I emailed it to myself and printed it.

These days, everything was taking me three times longer than it should. By the time I finished my log, prepared breakfast and lunch and got dressed, it was six o'clock. Time to get up.

Yossel drove me to my appointment, and before long the verdict was in. I needed bunion surgery.

"How am I going to walk after the surgery when my brain is already telling my legs not to walk?" I asked Yossel as we waited for the nurse to schedule the surgery.

"The bunion problem is not going to go away," he told me. "It will only get worse. You should have the operation as soon as possible. By the time the summer comes you'll be able to walk again." He watched as the door opened to admit another patient. "Every second person I've been speaking to knows someone who went through that surgery."

"And what do they say? Is it a breeze?"

"No, it's a little painful."

"Wow, that sure makes me feel better," I grumbled. "It's going to be so much easier now that I know that!"

We scheduled the surgery for April 20, right after Pesach and a few days after my birthday. I wondered if Berel and Sorah Rochel would still be in the United States, or if they'd have returned to Eretz Yisrael by then.

I signed the paper. I was one foot away from surgery.

Next stop: Dr. Fahn.

Over time, he'd been using the process of elimination to figure out what was wrong with me. Something was making me dizzy. Either it was the sickness itself or the medication I was taking to treat it. If my heart was fine and my bladder was fine, then maybe it was not MSA, after all. I'd been taking Azilect, a very expensive pill, on a daily basis. My friend Gittie Ryback was able to get that pill for me at no cost, through contacts in Eretz Yisrael.

Dr. Fahn decided that his next move would be to take me off the Azilect. He said it would be a few days before I'd see a change. If there was going to be one.

Within a day or two, I already saw a difference. I felt as if a cloud had been lifted from my head and I could think straight again. My blood pressure returned to normal; I checked it regularly. My speech was much clearer, and my balance was much improved. Overall, I felt better than I had in a long time.

"You look great!" one neighbor remarked.

"You look much better since I saw you last," a friend said when she met me.

"You're speaking so much more clearly!" my cousin mentioned when we spoke on the phone.

Everyone I saw commented on how great I looked and sounded. The dizziness was gone. I was able to step off the sidewalk without feeling as if the floor was moving under me or swaying from side to side. I was able to cross the street again, as I could once again turn my head to look both ways without the world spinning around. I could step up on the curb without losing my balance, and I could carry my pocketbook with me while I walked down the stairs. These things that we all take for granted every single day had become priceless treasures for me, and I was thrilled that I had gotten them back. It felt so much better that we canceled the bunion surgery.

Everyone who had been davening for me felt that Hashem had heard their prayers and helped me. I had to admit I felt that way, too. Hashem can change everything for the better in a blink of an eye.

But it didn't last.

As time went by, I began to notice the dizziness slowly creeping back. I was losing my balance again and could no longer cross the street on my own. At first, I refused to believe it. I was so disappointed and so scared. I took my blood pressure again: 98/72. Had it changed when I stood up? Was it fluctuating again?

Yossel and I had been so happy about the improvement in my condition. Yossel kept telling everyone, "Shami's much better!" Now it was all about to blow up in our faces. I told him that I was not feeling well, but he didn't want to hear it. Maybe, just then, he couldn't hear it.

In February, I had decided to attend a *sheva berachos* my cousin Debbie was giving for her nephew in honor of his marriage. I hadn't made it to the wedding itself, which was in the Marina Del Rey. It was just too far to travel, and the trip would have been too much for me. I'd stopped even attempting to attend such weddings.

At the party, all was going well. I sat down and spoke with my neighbors at the table in a higher pitch so that they could hear me. I got up and switched seats, trying to get comfortable. People were beginning to notice.

And then I started moving.

I felt everyone staring at me as I wiggled in my seat. The involuntary movements intensified. I had to get out of there. No one understood that the spasms build up and up, taking over your body until they totally absorb you.

I made it out of the room and had barely heaved a sigh of relief when I saw a few of the other guests following me out to see if I was okay. They thought I was hot and feeling faint. They were right. I knew I had to leave. Fast.

My sister carried my pocketbook, coat and make-up bag in one arm while she supported me with the other. She led me to a bench to wait for Yossel to bring the car around.

I was fuming with frustration and despair. I'd just finished telling everyone that the doctor had taken me off Azilect and that I was feeling better. I'd been telling my family and friends that I was not dying. I did not have Multiple System Atrophy. I did not have MSA!

I trembled, remembering how I'd recently told Yossel excitedly, "I do not have to say good-bye to all my family and friends. I do not have to give away all my personal possessions if I don't want to. The dizziness is much better. I'm seeing straight again!"

My emotions kept going up and down like a roller-coaster. They soared to the heights each time there was a glimmer of improvement, and plunged to the depths when the symptoms returned. As I sat on that bench waiting for my husband to take me home, I kicked myself for having such a big mouth. If I hadn't told everyone every detail of my sickness, the whole thing would have been easier to handle. Why had I been fine when I went off the medicine if everything now felt like it was caving in?

On my next visit to Dr. Fahn's office, Dr. Rothstein, his fellow, did the preliminary exam. Afterward, the doctors stood outside the doorway, speaking in low tones. They were discussing my case. I had a feeling I knew what they were saying, even though I didn't actually hear them.

"She's dizzy again," I imagined Dr. Rothstein reporting. "When I asked her to close her eyes and stand in one place, she started swaying. She has no balance. When I asked her to put one foot in front of the other, she keep touching the wall for support. When I took her blood pressure, it was 110/60 sitting down and dropped down to 85/60 when she stood up. I checked her heartbeat. It was irregular. Her heart skipped a beat after every fifth beat. She could not get up from the chair, and she falls back too fast when she sits down. When I pulled her back by the shoulders, she had to take five steps to catch her balance." And so on. I knew the score.

The doctors came back into the room. I was frightened.

Quickly, I explained to Dr. Fahn that when Dr. Rothstein examined me, it was an hour before I was due for my next dose of medicine. It was now fifteen minutes before the next dose was due.

"Maybe," I said hopefully, "that was why I couldn't get up easily from the chair or why I took too many steps back when he pulled me by the shoulders."

Dr. Fahn listened attentively as usual. I described my involuntary motions to him.

"You're anxious, Mrs. Reinman," he said. "I'm going to prescribe anti-anxiety pills."

"But the dyskinesia happens all the time." I told him that simply talking was such an effort that it made me tired and that's when I began to move around. In fact, the same thing is happening right now, as I type these words.

He still insisted that it was anxiety. He wrote out the prescription for anxiety pills.

The doctor wasn't wrong. I was anxious.

But then, after everything that had been happening to me, didn't I have good reason to be?

Health Kinesiology

There are many routes to good health. Apart from my visits to traditional doctors and the medications they prescribed for me, I had been ready and willing to try anyone or anything that sounded reasonable. The health kinesiologist was a frum Jew I had contacted even before Dr. Adams gave his diagnosis.

The first time I visited his home, he asked me for my full Hebrew name. I gave it to him: Shlomtza bas Chanah Sara. I sat at his dining-room table, my feet not touching the floor. Each time I came to his house after that first visit, he went through the same routine.

First, he gave me some sponge building blocks to place under my feet, and a towel to put behind my back to enable me to get comfortable. Then he lifted the lids of two cigar boxes full of glass tubes. Each glass tube had a different-colored coil inside.

He ran his fingers along the coils to see which one he was going to choose.

His middle finger rested on his index finger of his left hand, and his fingers were in constant motion, moving either up or down depending on my body's reaction to the question. If the answer was yes, the index finger could not be pushed down. If it was no, the left index finger was pushed down easily.

He placed one coil on himself and touched his shoe to my shoe so he could sense my energy. He handed me a coil and told me to place it on my thyroid, then another one to place on my navel. One day, he gave me coils for my head and back as well. My back had been hurting lately, but I hadn't said a word about it.

He told me there was bad energy coming from my computer and gave me a bead to put near it.

"Now, place four fingers on your thyroid, the front of the neck, and four fingers on the back of your neck, opposite your thyroid."

I couldn't reach the back of my neck.

He wrote, "fears/embarrassment," and told me to think about those two words. "Think about any traumatizing incident that happened when you were younger." Let me explain. In my mid-thirties I had had surgery for the removal of a melanoma. In addition in my early thirties I had been diagnosed with a tumor in the thyroid. It was a devastating experience, but b"H all went well and I recovered fully. The kinesiologist was referring to that episode.

"Think about the thyroid surgery and the melanoma," he instructed.

"I sometimes wonder why I didn't feel anything in my throat," I said. "After all, it was as large as a plum. I went to Eretz Yisrael with stitches in my throat for midwinter vacation. It wasn't easy."

He encouraged me to keep talking.

"The first thing that came to mind when I found the melanoma was: why did I wait so long? Why didn't I realize how dangerous it could be? A melanoma does not get bigger. It gets deeper and can kill a person very quickly. I was the head lifeguard; I should have known how dangerous the sun is. I had a responsible summer job, but after they did the biopsy I couldn't swim any more that summer." I rambled on.

The next time, he wrote, "dream; intimidated; recognizing."

"Do you want very much to dream about your grandmother, your father and your mother?" he asked.

"My husband dreamed about my mother and Bobby," I said. "In his dream, my mother said, 'Tell Bobby they aren't ready for her yet.'"

The next time, he wrote, "People with long-suffering illnesses."

"My neighbor," I said. "She lives on my block. She is in a wheelchair and cannot walk at all. I could use her wisdom, her strength and her wonderful insight. She is a brilliant woman. I would like to get to know her better. I don't visit her often enough."

"I want you to go home and smell alfalfa sprouts for 21 seconds, wait 5 seconds, and then again for 20 seconds."

This was getting weirder and weirder.

"What happened to you when you were three that was very traumatic?" he said. "Think about these ages. Think backward. What happened to you at the age of 58, 45, 25, 9 and 3?"

I couldn't think of anything.

He told me I was insecure. "Is it true that it's not easy for you to ask for help?"

I don't think that statement was true.

He kept talking and talking, and then suddenly, he stopped. "I'm sorry," he said. "I can't continue now. You have the mark of a big *ayin hara* on you. I'm going to call a rabbi to come over. He'll help you get rid of the *ayin hara*."

He pulled out his cell phone, and before I knew it, the rabbi was entering the house. Though small in stature, the rabbi looked very important as he walked in. He placed his hand on the kinesiologists', and they mumbled a few words back and forth. Sometimes, the kinesiologists's arm remained strong and horizontal, and at other times it went down. All this time, his shoe was touching my shoe.

The rabbi who had come to rid me of any *ayin hara* then told me in a British accent, "You have an *ayin hara* on you. But don't worry. I'll help you remove it."

He took a printed prayer from his pocket and began reciting. He went on reciting for a long time. I also noticed that he continued trying to press down the kinesiologists' arm.

Wow, I thought. This must be a serious *ayin hara* if he just keeps reading and reading. Later, I learned that this prayer must be said nine times.

He finally finished. They both yawned, and the kinesiologists' arm did not go down anymore.

The rabbi turned to me. "Is there someone who bears you a grudge, someone from whom you should ask forgiveness?"

I thought about it but came up empty.

"I want you to create an imaginary wall around you that no one can penetrate," the rabbi said. "I'll help you."

I tried to imagine a glass wall that I could see through. I poured sand, creating a glass rectangle in my mind, until I'd erected a protective wall all around myself.

"Make sure you seal it on top and on bottom so no one and nothing can penetrate it," he instructed. "The wall is good for nine months."

I wondered how I was supposed to breathe if it was sealed top and bottom.

"What if someone didn't forgive me," I said, "even though they said they did?"

"I want you to think about that person every morning. Think about loving that person for five minutes. After a while, that person will come around and truly forgive you."

"I'll try that."

By the time I left, I was exhausted.

Kinetic energy and *ayin haras*. Where else would my desperation lead me? Was there any hope for me?

Inner Strength

Devora hired a young woman from Grenada to help me in the house. Her name is Sadie Span, and when I first met her, she was all of twenty-one. I was apprehensive at first. It was embarrassing to show myself in all my weakness and let her do many of the things I wasn't able to do myself. But Sadie turned out to be a lifesaver. She was caring, understanding and a fun companion. She knew when I needed help and when I didn't want to be fussed over. Though she worried about me, she followed my cues.

The best thing was that she drove. I was mobile again! I no longer had to ask people to take me places. Sadie drove me to my appointments and stuck around if I needed help at activities. She saw me in both my good hours and my bad ones. Sadie was a pleasure to have around.

One day in January 2009, Sadie came with me to a meeting of a support group in Manalapan, a nearby town, just to see what it was like. I walked in late, because we'd lost our way. Most of the others there were old men and their female caregivers. I was the youngest in the room. And the one who had the most trouble walking.

The meeting took place on President Obama's Inauguration Day, and the group had decided to watch the ceremony on the Internet before I got there. By the time I arrived, they were rushing to catch up with the meeting's agenda. I can't say that I got much out of that meeting — except for one thing: aqua therapy. Everyone in the room raved about it.

"What exactly is it?" I wanted to know.

One elderly gentleman tried to describe it to me. "There's a treadmill in the water and a therapist to guide you." His eyes lit up. "You really must try it!"

Water therapy was an entirely different experience from the water aerobics I so enjoyed at the gym. I went down to Freehold, to view the facilities. I saw a small room with a small pool with a treadmill in the middle. It looked inviting enough. I made an appointment to try it.

On Wednesday morning, April Fool's Day, I had my first aqua therapy session.

Unfortunately, it was no joke.

Using the treadmill was harder than it looked. It took me quite a while to get myself moving on it. Tracy, the therapist, had me walk forward in the water for five minutes. That wasn't so bad, until I had to walk backward for the same length of time. The treadmill was going too fast for me. Before I knew it, my legs had floated up in the water, and I was holding onto the balancing bars for dear life!

The treadmill rolled serenely on without me. Tracy slowed it down. She had me walk forward and sideways as we watched my progress on a video screen.

"Kick sideways fifteen times... Kick back fifteen times... Go up and down on your heel fifteen times... Go up and down the step fifteen times... Now do the same with your left foot."

It all sounded great until I realized that there was no place to hold on. How in the world can they offer aqua therapy without handicap bars that an invalid can hold on to? I complained to the therapist. She told me to grip the ledge. I tried that and found it very difficult. The ledge was much too high for someone who is off-balance and only five feet tall. (The next session, I used a sponge noodle. That was better.)

I could hear music blasting from the room next door where they were doing aerobics at ninety miles an hour, while I was slipping and sliding, trying to get out of the pool. I had once been a lifeguard who used to do one hundred laps a day in the summer camp. Now I could barely stand in the water. As for swimming, it was a thing of the past.

"You should really use a rollator or walker when you walk outside," Tracy told me. "That's much better than using someone else for support."

"Why?" I asked.

"When you walk holding on to your friend's elbow," she explained, "she is setting the pace. Your brain is forgetting how to set a pace and will eventually forget how to walk."

I could not make my peace with that. Every time I thought about moving around outdoors with a walker, I cringed. I wasn't ready to make that transition. Anyway, shouldn't I wait until Shulem got married? Would it be fair to him to have people saying his mother was an invalid?

By the time I finished that first half-hour session, I could no longer move. I mean that literally. My mind was fuzzy, and I was seeing through a fog. My brain was asleep.

Two good friends came to visit me later, but I couldn't even join in the conversation. I had that sluggish, drowsy kind of feeling, as if I had been drugged. I could see that my lethargy was making them uncomfortable, and they kept eying each other, waiting for the moment when they could leave graciously.

I headed to bed to rest for a few minutes, and that helped to clear my mind. But by then, my friends were long gone.

Meanwhile, I was taking the anti-anxiety pills the doctor had prescribed, but I found that they were wearing off too quickly. If I took one every time I moved around, I'd be living on those pills. So I continued to search for new and effective therapies.

Rita Heap was the new addition to my list of therapists. A friend recommended that I see her for an ancient art of harmonizing body, mind and spirit through gentle touch. It's meant to facilitate balance in the body's energy systems, to promote health and well-being. Reading up on this "treatment" before my first appointment, I learned that it considers itself a supplement to conventional healing methods, inducing relaxation, reducing the effects of stress and assisting the body's capacity for healing.

All disease begins with blockages of energy, they say, and a person's pulse shows the practitioner the specific energy points that need to be pressed to restore a harmonious flow without creating additional stress in the patient's mind about her condition.

Rita claimed to see that my energy was blocked in certain places; pressing on an opposing part of the body at the same time would release the bad energy and allow fresh energy to flow. Sadie usually came with me and was learning how to do it.

"Did anything happen to you right before you got sick?" Rita Heap asked.

I find it very interesting that most of those who have tried to help me have asked that question. I told her about the deaths of my parents with whom I was very close. She actually gave me an exercise to do while thinking about them. "This will help you grieve," she said.

Another project I kept busy with was creating collages and preparing pictures to hang on the wall. Even though I felt crummy, I was not ready to stop being the active person I had always been. I hated the feeling of not being in control of my own body. Often, I felt as though the rest of the world was floating at a distance.

Every doctor I saw asked me, "Are you depressed?"

"I'm not depressed," I told them. "I'm just sad that I'm not well."

"You're not in touch with your emotions," one of them told me. "Wake up! You have a serious disease. You are experiencing pain, both mentally and physically."

If all this was hard for me, it was a nightmare for Yossel. As soon as it became clear that this was a permanent condition, he began retreating. He just didn't know how to deal with the new reality. He started spending most of the night writing in his office, staying there for longer and longer periods of time.

Everything was going downhill, except for my weight. When I walked around the block two times with a neighbor or a friend, it felt as if I were lifting a couple of tree trunks instead of my legs. I begged to go back home.

"Don't talk about your sickness all day," my husband told me one evening. "That's all you talk about. Eventually, people will start staying away."

He was right, of course, and I knew it. Though my illness absorbed me, it was difficult for other people to deal with. They needed me to be the best Shami that I could be. So I suppressed my feelings and my fears. My body would have to find the strength and spirit to overcome what was afflicting it. I had to be stronger than the situation.

Inner strength, that's what I needed. How was I going to find some?

I found some relief in writing down my thoughts.

> I'm so tired of fighting. I'll fight tomorrow. Tomorrow will be a better day. I need support, an infusion of strength from my family, friends and neighbors. I can't do this alone.
>
> I'm trying to be strong, but how can I be in control of a situation that I don't really control? I try to laugh and smile, but my face shows no expression. I place my hands on my chest and take deep, cleansing breaths. If I don't do that, my breathing becomes very shallow. What if I'm forgetting how to breathe?
>
> I must daven to Hashem, because He is the only One Who can help me. I say some *Tehillim*, because that is supposed to be therapeutic. But my lips don't form the words properly. I find myself using my eyes to read, not my lips. I try to focus, but the words do not behave.

The beginnings and ends of the words appear unusually light. It's hard for me to focus,

Opening a box is painful. I have to do it ever so slowly. I have to do a lot of things slowly. My mind is so cloudy, but I want to do it all now, while I can still think.

At the table, I want to say something, but it's such an ordeal that I procrastinate. I finally manage to say it, but no one hears me. Then the shushing starts. By the time everyone quiets down so they can make sure I am heard, the comment I was going to say is not nearly as important or interesting. I feel so stupid.

The meal is over. I tried to get up from my chair, but my brain is ignoring me. I don't move. I slowly rock back and forth, to gain momentum. Finally, I'm on my feet, but they seem glued to the floor. My guests are going out the door. I can't get to them in time to see them off. I call out good-bye, but they don't hear me. They are gone.

Writing helped, but I knew that I had to find an even higher level of acceptance and trust in Hashem. To recognize that even these difficult years are valuable and beautiful. To pull out a smile when I felt more like crying.

To remember that all of life is so precious. Even the most painful parts.

Mrs. Reinman's Disease

My toes had been giving me a lot of grief. It's amazing, how much we take those little things called toes for granted. We expect them to keep us upright and to take us where we want to go. But from the beginning, even before I was diagnosed with Parkinson's, my toes had refused to cooperate.

After years of pain and visits to the doctor, it had been decided that I would definitely need bunion surgery even though I had canceled the first surgery. But first, I went to get Botox shots on my toes in Columbia Presbyterian. Dr. Pullman would only do one foot. He said my body couldn't take too much and if both feet received the treatment it would take away my balance. Instead, he administered two cortisone shots to the two middle toes on my right foot.

At home, I settled down to watch bunion surgery on my computer. It never ceases to amaze me that I can get all the information I need about anything without ever leaving my house.

The video was pretty scary. A girl with bright red nail polish on her toes was undergoing surgery. She was sitting on an upright table, pillows behind her head, watching as the bone of her big toe was being shaved off. Yikes! It sounded like the drill in a dentist's office.

I called my family to tell them about my upcoming operation.

"I went to a surgeon's office ..." Inevitably, at this point, whoever I was talking to would exclaim, "A surgeon! Of course a surgeon is going to say you need surgery!"

"I talked it over first with my Parkinson's doctor," I explained again and again, "and he told me, 'You can do the surgery; you're strong enough to snap back.'"

But my relatives were skeptical, and I was nervous. So I went to see my primary physician, Dr. Eddie Santiago, to tell him how I felt about the surgery. I'd been recommended to Dr. Santiago by Dr. Howard Lebowitz, who runs an acute-care facility in Lakewood. I'd been told that he was very knowledgeable and caring and that I should definitely try to see him.

I tried for two years. Dr. Lebowitz doesn't see outpatients; he works solely in the hospital. I called repeatedly, trying to get an appointment. Finally, he spoke to me on the phone. "I'm sorry," he said, letting me down gently. "I can't see you. I don't treat outpatients." And then he recommended his student, Dr. Santiago.

Dr. Santiago has an office in Deal, New Jersey. Stepping inside, I found myself surrounded by about fifty other patients. There were various medical personnel milling around, and Yossel and I spent the half-hour wait trying to figure out which one was the doctor and which were his assistants.

At last, it was my turn to go inside. Dr. Santiago looks like a roly-poly Hispanic kid. After meeting him, I felt very secure. He was brilliant, and I felt that he understood me. The office was always very busy, but I was able to communicate with him via texting. In this way, I could order prescriptions and have my questions answered.

Dr. Santiago was the one who'd taken care of me in the hospital when I had an infection. Now, as I faced my bunion dilemma,

I decided to get his advice about the surgery. The arguments for and against kept going through my mind until I was even dizzier than usual. To operate, or not to operate? That was the question.

I sat facing the doctor and explained the situation. "The surgeon says if I don't do the surgery now the bunion will only get worse. It is pushing my other four toes to the side, making me lose my balance and fall easily."

Dr. Santiago considered this, and nodded. "Better you should do it now and not wait until you are worse."

Taking a deep breath, I told him how I felt about the post-operative period. I didn't think that I could go home directly after the surgery. I felt that being home and on my own would simply overwhelm me. "I feel so weak all the time. I can't see myself being self-sufficient at home."

He saw my point and offered to help me set up something for after the surgery. He called his friend, a doctor in Acute Rehab. The friend agreed to accept me for three days of acute care, followed by a convalescent period in a nursing home. I could sign up with Leisure Chateau, a facility in Lakewood.

It all sounded perfect. There was just one problem. Dr. Santiago would have to call my insurance plan first to get their permission.

The good doctor went to a lot of trouble for me. He stayed on the phone with Blue Cross Blue Shield for a full fifty minutes. In the end, however, he was unsuccessful. My insurance refused to cover the stay.

In retrospect, this was a blessing, because I was getting more apprehensive as each day brought me closer to the surgery.

"Calm down," everyone told me.

But the calmer they were, the more terrified I became.

And then, out of the blue, my brother-in-law Sruli called us up and said that Dr. Lebowitz was willing to see us. It turned out that he and his family were huge fans of the books my husband had written as Avner Gold.

Dr. Lebowitz lives in Lakewood, and we met him in his private study at home. Yossel and he instantly hit it off and have since become very good friends. Before discussing the bunion, we gave him the background on my situation. I launched into an explanation of my situation and the emotions surrounding it. I told him that my doctor could not decide conclusively if I had Parkinson's or MSA.

"Neurological diseases come in many different forms," he said. "They can resemble one kind of disease or another or more than one. If you want to attach a name to what you have I would call it Mrs. Reinman's disease."

What an honor. I could have a disease named after me.

"The question we have now is this," I said. "I've been urged to have bunion surgery, and Dr. Santiago agrees that it's probably a good idea. But I just don't feel I should be off of my feet for a year if it could be MSA and my time might be limited."

I looked at the doctor anxiously, awaiting his verdict.

To my surprise, he agreed with me. "Anything that could go wrong will probably go wrong. You'd become a perfect candidate for being the kind of acutely-ill patient I deal with full time." He leaned forward. "Unless you are in excruciating pain from the bunion, do not have the surgery."

My sigh of relief could be heard all the way to the other side of the house.

"Call me any time you need my help," Dr. Lebowitz said graciously, and he gave us his private cell number.

He'd made up my mind for me. I was going to put up with the pain in light of my larger and much more pressing goal of living each day to the fullest.

As time went on, the friendship between Yossel and Dr. Lebowitz deepened. They would spend many hours together discussing all kinds of topics, from Chumash and Gemara to philosophy, science and politics, and I could see clearly that they thoroughly enjoyed each other's company.

True to his word, Dr. Lebowitz has been coming to see me in my house right away whenever I need him. And he responds immediately to our numerous emails and texts. I know that Hashem has put me in the best hands, and I am deeply grateful.

Laughter Therapy

Purim is a day tailor-made for forgetting your problems. It's a day for dressing up, for gorging on sweets, for sending elaborate food packages to friends and neighbors. It's a time to put aside our cares and troubles while remembering the great miracle Hashem performed for the Jewish people on that long-ago Purim in Persia.

Queen Esther I'm not, but I believe in miracles, too. That Purim, I decided to celebrate with a "walkerthon."

In keeping with the medical theme, I bought candy canes, prunes, winkies — because they look like pills — surgical gloves, granny apples and a pill box to fill my gift baskets. When they were done, they looked adorable.

I dressed up as a granny with a gray-haired wig. The whole neighborhood came to check it out. I never ended up using the walker at all that Purim. I just wanted to be a "bobby," a grandmother. This is the poem I wrote for the occasion.

Send them to Granny

You might look in every nook and cranny
For someone loving like you,
You may need your very own nanny
Just to lend you a hand or two.
You can always count on dear old granny,
She's the one who'll pull you through.

Granny will keep your kids well fed,
Whenever they come over.
A place where they can relax their heads,
They'll never get tired of her.

She'll even put them to bed,
Send pajamas, no pillow or cover.
She'll play games, they'll be well read.
And the kids will always love her.

Love, Shami (Bobby) Reinman

They say that laughing is wonderful therapy. In that vein, Rochel Marder, whom I met through Devora, is a professional laughter therapist. She's a genuine comedienne who goes to hospitals, nursing homes and people's homes just to bring laughter into people's lives.

One night in January 2009, the doorbell rang. I opened the door, and in swam Rochel Marder, all dressed and ready for the pool. She wore flippers on her feet, a bathing cap with a wig underneath, a snorkel and goggles. I played along with her act and Devora videotaped it. What a comedy! For a few minutes, I forgot all about my issues.

Another time, she came to my house dressed as a bag lady and performed a hilarious skit for me and my friends. We all laughed until tears rolled down our faces.

I mentioned to Rochel once that I was experiencing pain in my toes. The next thing I knew, she was sitting in my house wearing enormous red toes on her feet!

She's created her own CD, which she hands out whenever

she hears that someone can use a laugh. After I watched it, I was literally chuckling for a good half-hour.

Now, more than ever, I find myself irresistibly drawn to people who have the gift of laughter. My grandson Berel, Devora's second son, also loves to make people laugh. When he was younger, he used to dress up at every opportunity. It was hilarious. Berel is a tremendous help to me. He is very affectionate, and there is a deep connection between us. In many ways, he is similar to me, and he gets me. He is very inquisitive and tenacious, and we've spent many pleasurable hours working on projects together or playing games. He visits me all the time, and even from yeshivah, he never fails to call and check on me. When I get off the phone with him, there is always a big smile on my face.

Tzvi, my one and only son-in-law, Devora's husband, is another wonderful source of laughter for me. When he sees me start to spasm or lose my balance, he cracks a good one-liner and defuses the entire situation. When I lost my balance and tripped, he said, "Mom, stop dancing in the street and get into the car." He knows how to make me laugh. He's also always there for me; whenever I need something, he'll come running. When I showed him this book, he told me to save him for the sequel.

One evening, Rochel and I decided to frame all the collages and pictures I'd created that year. Rochel promised to hang them on the walls for me. To get the supplies we needed, she took me to Wal-Mart, where I drove one of those handicap carts for the first time. I didn't mind as much as I'd thought I would, because I was focused on the project. Hanging all of my collages and the many pictures of my children and grandchildren was not going to be an easy task.

Over the next few nights, my collages and pictures were framed and hung to decorate my walls. Putting six extra holes in the wall was certainly worth it. Rochel was off the wall, and I was having a ball!

My daughter, at age thirty-six, had gone back to school in September 2007 to train as a social worker. During those years, her children practically lived in my house whenever she had to attend classes. We got involved in many projects. Being a loving grandmother does not take much physical effort. The kids didn't care if I could talk or walk. They sang their songs and danced for me, and I was a great audience, full of love and admiration for them.

One Sunday, we came up with a surprise plan. We decided to produce a video for Devora, featuring her four girls: Batsheva, Blimi, and Raizy and Chanala, the twins, who'd be turning five that month. The whole thing was top secret, a Mother's Day surprise for my daughter.

The original idea was for them to just sing a Mom song, but as I looked around for songs I found two others I wanted to try. As soon as the twins heard the songs they wanted to sing them. So they ended up singing three songs: the Mom song, "I Am the Cute One," and "Identical Twins."

Since we were babysitting for the twins while Devora was in school, they had a lot of time to practice. Batsheva and Blimi practiced with them for four solid months. And through those entire four months, the twins managed to keep the secret. Every time they walked into the house, I would have the songs playing on my laptop. They complained to me, "We don't want to go to Bobby's house. All we do is practice!"

Batsheva, who is very artistic, drew signs. We borrowed some hats, went to the Dollar Store for costumes and dressed the twins up. Then we videotaped them singing. The video came out so good that whoever came into the house watched it. A proud Bobby, I also emailed it to everyone I knew.

As for Devora, she was so surprised and moved that for a long time after that special Mother's Day she watched that video three times a day.

Almost Drowning

In July 2009, I traveled to Manhattan again to see Dr. Fahn. It had been four months since my previous visit. Dr. Fahn changes fellows just about every year. As soon as I get used to the fellow, a new one appears. This time the fellow was Dr. Sheng Kuo, who had a slight accent and a round face with typically Oriental features.

I always meet the fellow first to discuss my case and any new symptoms that may have crept up on me since my previous visit. I met Dr. Kuo in one of the examining rooms.

He took my blood pressure. “120/70. Perfect!”

I stood up, and he took my pressure again. This time, it was 95/60. Significantly lower.

The door opened and in walked Dr. Fahn with two visiting doctors close behind. I think one was from Spain and the other from Eretz Yisrael. He examined me and began asking questions. As soon as I started to speak, the dyskinesia woke up. My right shoulder began jerking, my head started shaking, and then my neck, jaw and right thigh joined in. After that the right side of my mouth began to pull down.

"I see that the dyskinesia begins when you start talking," Dr. Fahn observed.

"No wonder it's a problem," I said. "I talk a lot!"

Everyone laughed.

"Dr. Fahn, did you know that I'm writing a book?" I asked.

"What about?"

"About my life and what happened to me. And you're in it." I watched his reaction out of the corner of my eye. He looked quite interested.

"I'll give you a copy when it's done," I promised.

"I'll be very interested to read it."

Dr. Fahn turned to address the three doctors in the room with us. "Why does the dyskinesia start on the right side, where the Parkinson's is?"

My husband piped up. "It goes to where the medicine is."

Dr. Fahn turned to Yossel. "I'm not asking you. I'm asking Dr. Sheng Kuo and these two doctors. But you're right!"

I'd made a list of new symptoms, or symptoms that had become worse since my last appointment. I handed it to Dr. Fahn.

Dr. Fahn gave me a stronger sleeping pill and upped the dosage on my Selegeline. He told me to get an MRI of my shoulder. My other orders were to take speech therapy, do exercise and see an ENT doctor and an eye doctor. Being a Parkinson's patient is a full-time job!

Later that night, I sat in front of my computer and typed the day's entry.

> Today is a fast day, the seventeenth day of Tammuz, the day the walls of Jerusalem were breached after a long siege that led to its destruction thousands of years ago. I am not fasting. With all the medication I'm taking, I was told not to fast even on Yom Kippur.

Here was yet another way my illness was taking me away from the routines and rituals I loved. Not that I loved fasting on Yom Kippur. But I loved what refraining from eating and drinking for twenty-five hours did for me. Leaving the body behind for an entire day frees you to finally feel your soul. The day I was told never to fast again was a sad one for me.

On Friday night, we were invited to have our meal at the home of my friend Yvette Cohen. I did not realize that all her sisters, brothers, sisters-in-law and brothers-in-law would also be there as well. It would have been fine if I'd been feeling well, but Dr. Fahn had just switched my medications. The spasms started gradually, but they grew worse and worse as the night wore on. Finally, I had to beg to go home.

I rested up over Sunday. Monday morning, my friend Chaya and I were invited to my friend Raizy's Olympic-size pool. Raizy Yurowitz and I have been friends for many years. I had given her refresher courses in First Aid and CPR through the years. I taught her computers, and she taught me WSI and refreshed my lifeguarding course. Before I contracted Parkinson's disease, I'd been a devoted and energetic swimmer. Now, afraid of losing my balance I avoided swimming, but she'd been asking me to come for quite a while. So I went.

I was walking in the shallow end of the pool holding on to a sponge noodle for extra balance when I started to float.

"Help!" I shouted. "I'm floating up!"

"That's good," she answered, not realizing I was in trouble.

"I can't get down!" I yelled as I started to fall back. "I'm drowning!"

Chaya realized this was no joke and came to my rescue. She helped me stand up, and I just stood there holding onto her and gasping for breath. I'd had enough.

A few days later, Leah Trenk drove me to the Catskills. Leah and I go way back. She was my counselor when I was a camper many years ago, the assistant principal when I taught in Ilan, and a wonderful friend to me to this very day. I went to visit my sister who was working in a camp. I watched a play rehearsal and walked into the dining room for meals holding on to my sister's arm. In the evening, my sister and our cousin took me out for dinner. On the way home, we must have driven over fifteen speed bumps. I think that's what finally did me in.

That night, my right rib started hurting again. The pain became worse and worse as the night went on. By morning, I groaned with every breath. I was supposed to stay in camp for a week, but I was in such pain that I couldn't settle down or enjoy anything. I finally got a ride home in a van that was not meant for human transportation.

Dr. Lebowitz was kind enough to come over to our house to check on me. He gave me codeine, but it had little effect. He came again on Sunday night. He asked me if I would be relieved to know that I was going to be hospitalized. I said, truthfully, that I was. I just wanted to be rid of the pain.

We decided I would check myself into the hospital on Tuesday morning so I wouldn't have to go in during the night. Dr. Lebowitz said I would be going in for pain management, which basically meant morphine through an intravenous line. An X-ray was taken, to see if my rib was broken. It wasn't.

Finally, after almost continuous pain until Wednesday afternoon, the orthopedist came in and gave me an injection right into the muscle. I felt a little better, so they sent me home.

A few days later, my friend Yvette asked if I wanted to go to the mall with her to buy a pair of slippers. I told her I could only get around in a wheelchair, but I didn't want to visit any of the malls in our vicinity because I might meet people who knew me. I wasn't ready for that yet.

When Devora called, I told her that I'd turned down the outing because I didn't want to go to the mall in a wheelchair. My daughter became very earnest and very firm.

"Mommy, you're just punishing yourself," she said. "You didn't do anything wrong! You're not allowing yourself to have any fun. You don't go out at all, you don't walk outside anymore, and it's not good for you. You're getting weaker and weaker."

She was making sense. In my fear of what people would say, I'd practically made myself housebound. I deserved to get out more. I wanted to get out more. And if it took being seen in public in a wheelchair, so be it!

Taking a deep breath, I called Yvette back to tell her that I'd changed my mind. But she was no longer home.

Here's an entry from that difficult week:

August 4, 2009

I feel my time is limited. I am not telling this to anyone. But my spasms have gotten much tighter and more painful. My balance is worse. I can barely walk and I'm extremely dizzy. I stopped walking outside.

Shulem has a date coming up. I don't even think I am capable of meeting a girl, let alone the parents of the girl.

But that is just today. Tomorrow may be better.

The Baby's Name

Interspersed with the down days, which were absorbed by fighting my symptoms and my fears, there were some definite high points. One of them was in June 2009, when Cindy and Chaim became the proud parents of another baby boy.

Yossel had asked Cindy several months earlier if she knew what she was having, a boy or a girl. She had answered with a twinkle in her eye, "I know what I'm having, but I'm not telling."

I visited Cindy in the hospital. She looked great. The baby was in the bassinet right next to her. He was beautiful. Whipping out my cell phone, I took a picture of him and set it as the phone's wallpaper. He was a darker version of his five-year-old brother, Eli. I held him in my arms for a few minutes, until my shoulders tired. Then I listened in shock as Cindy described her experience.

"The baby didn't breathe right away. They had to suction him. Finally, he gave a little whimper, and then he cried. The whole experience took about fifty seconds, but they were the longest fifty seconds of my life."

The story brought back old memories of Shulem, who'd been born nearly ten years after my previous child, Berel. When I was expecting, I was terrified that something would be wrong with him. As soon as he was born, I saw that he was blue and not breathing. The medical staff whisked him away. A minute later, which felt like forever, I heard him cry. What a beautiful sound! Shulem was fine.

And so, thank Hashem, was my beautiful grandson.

It was time to choose a name.

This was no simple decision in our family, since I was quite sensitive about the topic and could get pretty riled up when giving my opinion. Making my point took a lot of effort. Everyone was louder than I was those days, and not all of them agreed with me. However, I still insisted on stating my case.

In Jewish tradition, every grandparent's soul has a connection to the soul of the newborn baby that bears his or her name. In addition, there is also a connection to all the ancestors who had that name in earlier generations. And often, as the child grows up, it becomes apparent that he or she has some of the same traits and characteristics as the person for whom he or she is named. If parents avoid giving a particular name because they don't like it, that grandparent will be deprived of a connection to future generations.

For instance, my great-grandfather's name was Isamar Rosenbaum. He was a great man, and I was very close to him. However, my children didn't care for the name and didn't want to saddle a child with it. While I could understand that, I still felt that a name was important and should not just be left out of the running.

Sometimes I wondered: What if my sister had not started using the nickname Shami for me in place of my real name, Shlomtza? Would everyone have called me Shlomtza? Could I have lived with that name? Would my grandchildren want to give their babies that name after I left this world?

Yossel agrees with my children. If the baby's parents don't like a certain name, he believes, they should not have to use it for their child. Unless it is the name of a parent. Then there is the issue of honoring one's parents, and the question becomes more complicated. My granddaughter Batsheva is actually Batsheva Yenta, the second name after Yossel's mother, but she is known as Batsheva. That is a fair compromise.

"I'm not going to offer any opinion about what name to choose," he declared after Chaim and Cindy's baby was born.

As for me, here's what I would have liked to say to them: "I'm not going to tell you what to do. But if I were you, I would name the baby after my father."

I thought it over and realized that what was really bothering me was that it was so hard to voice my opinion on anything. The minute I'd start, there would be a heated discussion, and I wasn't capable of participating. That really bothered me.

I tried to explain to Cindy how I felt. "If you would hear me out, and then say, 'I'm sorry, but I just don't think I could give that name because...' then I would back down."

Cindy understood me. That felt good.

And then came something that made me feel even better. A few days before the *bris*, when a Jewish boy traditionally receives his name, Chaim told me that they'd decided to name the baby Esriel, after my father.

I hadn't felt so happy in a long, long time.

Just thinking about it makes the tears flow. And then the spasms. I wanted to thank Cindy and Chaim from the bottom of my heart for giving me the privilege and honor of watching this child, Esriel, grow up in their home.

Not long after that celebration, I was getting ready to mark another, very different one. My friend Chaya had just turned sixty-five. I wanted to do something meaningful for her birthday, and it had to be done before she went on vacation. After some thought, I decided to put together a video of our friendship and of our children growing up together. I knew this would mean a lot to her.

I set the video to a tune I knew she would love. "You Light Up My Life" was a song we used to listen to when the kids were younger. It was hard to believe we'd been friends for thirty-five years!

Devora looked through all her photo albums, and I looked through mine. We emailed the family and gathered whatever material we could find. Devora helped me with the program, and we worked feverishly to get it done on time. We finally finished the video on Friday morning. Chaya was leaving right after Shabbos.

On Friday afternoon, Devora called Chaya and told her to come over with her daughter, Mindy, ostensibly to cheer me up. The minute they walked into the house, we practically threw her into the recliner. The music started, and so did her tears. She had recognized the first few notes immediately and sat mesmerized as the video played.

Pictures of us dressed up as Raggedy Ann. Chaya giving the first haircut at age three to my son Chaim, who was now thirty-five. All the recent pictures I'd been snapping that week were in there. It was a pictorial celebration of Chaya's life and our friendship, lovingly wrapped in the music we both loved. Now she understood what had been going on right under her nose.

The video was a big hit. Chaya called me from the airport on Saturday night and told me, "All Shabbos, I was singing that tune over and over in my head. Thank you, Shami."

I felt as if it were I who should be thanking her for decades of the most devoted friendship in the world. Though some days I felt my life shrinking in on itself like an ever-narrowing tunnel, at that moment it seemed to expand until it was as wide as my joy. I felt blessed.

The Elephant in the Room

One day in that summer of 2009, I asked Yossel, "So how's the work going?" My husband usually has a number of projects going at once, but both of us knew exactly which one I meant. Mine.

I'd basically finished writing my book, though I kept adding bits and pieces to it every now and then. A friend of mine, Rochelle Gemal, had proofread the manuscript. She texted me the very next morning. "I didn't sleep all night. I can't believe what you went through. Your manuscript is warm and well written, and I feel sorry for you. I couldn't put it down!"

Now it was Yossel's turn. He'd recently completed a 150,000-word book that he'd been working on, and his time was somewhat freed up. Way back when he first suggested that I write down my experiences in book form, he'd made me a promise. I would write it, and he would edit it and rewrite whatever needed to be rewritten. I'd kept my part of the bargain, but Yossel was having a hard time keeping his.

He looked frustrated. "I'm trying, Shami. I really am. I sat down at my computer again this morning, determined to work on the book. But I found myself doing everything else instead."

"Why is it so hard?" I wondered aloud.

He shook his head. "You know I've done many books in other people's voices. I'm very good at it. But this is just too overwhelming. I feel this terrible pressure on me, because I want so much to do a good job for you. But it's just not working."

I very badly wanted my book to be finished, but at the same time it was clear that things couldn't go on as they were. I had an idea. "Why don't you take a little vacation? Recharge your batteries."

Yossel lit up.

We talked about it some more, and I suggested that he take Shulem with him on a week-long trip. Vacations were out of the question for me now. I had trouble just walking down the hall to my bed.

Yossel was torn. "Should I go? Shulem really wants to see Texas. This is the only time of year when he has no yeshivah. I really could use a vacation. But, really, I don't have to go. If you feel bad about it, I could just stay home."

I told him I didn't mind. I said I wanted him and Shulem to have a great time together. He must have caught a wistful note in my voice, though, because he said, "Maybe you can go somewhere, too. One of your friends could take you away for a day or two. Or maybe you could go to your sister."

Once again, Yossel was trying to make us both believe that my friendships could work as a substitute for my marriage. We both missed the companionship we'd shared before my illness. But at that point, I was the only one who was prepared to talk about it.

"Maybe," I said. "Meanwhile, you go ahead and make your plans. Why shouldn't you take a trip just because I can't?"

Yossel jumped into action. He phoned our cousins in New Orleans and made arrangements to go there for Shabbos. He and Shulem would spend the weekdays driving through Texas.

I did feel wistful, but I'd meant what I'd said. Why should my husband be homebound just because my ability to travel had become limited? Like I said, I'm a realist. Things are what they are. But it wasn't so much the prospect of being left behind when they went to Texas that bothered me. It was the fact that I felt as if I'd already been left behind in my own home.

For the past few months, when Yossel, Shulem and I sat down at the supper table, we'd made a joint decision not to answer the phone during the meal. In that way, we could hear about each other's days without interruption. Lately, however, I'd begun to realize that Yossel had been talking to only one person throughout the meal. And that person was not me.

On the nights Shulem went to school, supper would be over in a few minutes. It was hard for me to swallow and chew without choking. Yossel would tell me how much work was waiting for him, and then he'd return to his study. He would not come upstairs again until very late. I understood that my situation had put us under great financial pressure, and the burden fell squarely on Yossel's shoulders.

"I wish you could relax and spend more time with me," I would say.

"Maybe when I finish my book," he would usually say. He was referring to an exciting novel he'd been commissioned to write on a subject dear to his heart: proving that the Bible was a valid historical record. It was an ambitious project, and he'd already been at it for years. He'd had to go back and rewrite the book several times, and I knew it was consuming him. I also knew that he would not give up until he had succeeded.

I also think that there was a little more to it than just time pressure. Yossel couldn't take my spasms. He couldn't bear that I was sick. He couldn't bear that his beautiful wife had been reduced to an invalid wracked by spasms and dyskinesias. So he took refuge in his study and in his work.

I understood this as well. We'd had a rich, full life together before the Parkinson's came along. We'd been the best of friends, companions and travel partners. Now, Yossel didn't know what to do with the new me. He didn't know how to fit himself into the new reality, a reality that he'd never asked for and that he hated with every fiber of his being.

I hated it, too. But I'd been working hard, from day one, to come to terms with it. To strengthen my faith to meet the challenges that my worsening condition brought home to me on a daily basis. Yossel needed me to be the way I had been before. But I needed him to accept me the way I was now. It all came to a head one night when we finally talked about it. He told me he couldn't help it, and we both cried.

"What am I supposed to do?" Yossel said. "I feel like there's a big elephant in the room with us. This elephant follows us everywhere. You always talk about your sickness. You look like you're in pain most of the day. I don't blame you. I feel terrible for you. I know that if the tables were turned you would do much better than I'm doing. You would be an angel of mercy. But I just can't deal with it."

"So what am I supposed to do?" I asked in exasperation.

Even as I asked the question, I knew what Yossel's answer would be. Get dressed every day, put on some make-up and don't talk about it so much.

I'm a realist. If Yossel couldn't accept the situation, then it was up to me to do so. I decided that I'd better pull myself together and not wallow in self-pity, or I was going to lose out on the precious time I had left with my family.

I would plant a smile on my face and keep the tears right where they belonged.

Inside.

Group Prayers

My granddaughter Batsheva came over early one Shabbos morning to see if I needed help. We were having guests for the afternoon *seudah*. My dyskinesia was especially strong that morning, and Batsheva was concerned.

"Bobby, I've seen you moving before, but this is really unusual. Last week, when you were moving around, you told me it's just a side effect of the medications you're taking. But this doesn't look like a side effect! It looks much more serious. Unless you're just dancing to your own tune."

I guess that's what I'm doing. Dancing to a very personal tune that my body keeps making up as I go along. I did my best to reassure Batsheva. Soon afterward, our guests arrived. I welcomed them warmly and tried to be a gracious hostess, while working hard to suppress the involuntary movements that kept trying to take over. All in all, however, it was a pleasant meal.

That week, my friend Idy Yoffe told me that she'd arranged for a group of women to recite *Tehillim* for forty days using the letters of my name, Shlomtza bas Chanah Sara. She'd emailed my friends, neighbors, and relatives, all of whom were eager to participate. Each one would be responsible for reciting the particular chapter or chapters of *Tehillim* that corresponded to the letters of my Hebrew name. Idy told me to recite the last chapter myself to complete my name.

The massive prayer project would start that Sunday near the end of Av 2011 and end on the day before Rosh Hashanah, forty days in all. There is a special spiritual significance to prayers said for a specific purpose for forty consecutive days.

On Erev Yom Kippur, my friends got together in my daughter's house to bake *challos* together and then perform the mitzvah of taking *challah* as a group. Perhaps in the merit of this Jewish woman's holy mitzvah I would be granted a reprieve. I was also there and took part in the mitzvah. All in all, forty women came with their dough in their pans. Chanie Schwartz, the rebbetzin of our shul, opened the event with a short and beautiful speech that inspired us all with the significance of what we were doing. It was a very moving experience, and we've repeated it every year since.

Perhaps together we can change this terrible decree, I thought. The Chida, Rabbi Chaim Yosef Dovid Azoulai, a wise sage who lived in the 1700s, said that certain formulas in prayer can change a person's destiny. Maybe Hashem would hear all our prayers and bring about a speedy recovery for which we would all praise Him.

A few days later, my friend Raizy called me again to see if I would go swimming. As soon as I got up from my chair, I was dizzy.

"Maybe that's not such a good idea," I told her.

"But I heated the pool just for you!"

I felt a pang of guilt. "Okay," I said. "I'll try going again."

It took all my strength to walk across the room and get into my bathing suit. I spent about twenty minutes in the pool. I clung to the wall and kicked my legs, and then I walked across the shallow water a few times. I was moving. The water was moving. I was so dizzy.

I paid the price for my exertions the next day. In the morning, I couldn't turn my waist and my joints were stiff. I held my breath and moved through the pain that was ravaging my joints and side.

As usual, Cindy came to my assistance. She called the doctor and described my symptoms down to the last detail as well as anyone possibly could. He added Amantadine to my ever-growing list of medications. This was supposed to provide me with dopamine without the accompanying dyskinesia. The doctor explained that I would have to build up the dose until I was taking four pills a day.

Over the next few days, I saw an improvement. We put up railings in the bedroom along the whole wall to make it easier for me to get around the room. We also added a few more handicap grips in the bathroom.

I was doing a little better on the Amantadine. My family, friends and neighbors were davening for me. My spirits were a little higher.

Dreams and Hallucinations

One night, I saw Batsheva standing right beside my bed, and I said to her, "Would you please bring me a drink of water?" Yossel heard me and sat up in bed. He gave me a queer look.

"Who are you talking to?" he said.

I cleared my head and saw that there was no one there. I mumbled something, turned over and closed my eyes. I had seen someone who wasn't there. Was this the next step in my decline? Was I going to be seeing hallucinations all the time? Was I losing my mind? My greatest fear was always dementia. I wanted to finish my life with dignity and a clear mind. I was horrified at the prospect of becoming demented.

On another night, I saw a piece of flax in a sort of cylinder shape. It was moving gently back and forth, back and forth, right there in front of my eyes. Was this another hallucination? Maybe

I was dreaming. I sat up and rubbed my eyes. No, I was wide awake. This was no dream, but it looked very real.

The next night, I was screaming and crying in my sleep so loudly that I woke Yossel. He gently tried to wake me and calm me down. I was deep into my nightmare and couldn't pull myself so easily to the surface of consciousness. Yossel gently shook my shoulder, and I finally came awake.

"Shh, it's only a dream," he was saying soothingly. "Just calm down and go back to sleep. Only sweet dreams."

I went back to sleep, but pretty soon, I was screaming again.

The next day, I called the doctor and told him about my nightmares and hallucinations. It was a not uncommon side effect, he explained, of the Selegeline and Amantadine, the medications I was taking. It should get better over time. Well, that was a relief. At least I wasn't losing my mind.

Being a computer person, I found myself spending loads of time online, researching my medications and symptoms and looking for a ray of hope, any kind of a lifeline I could grasp. Among other things, I read about DBS, deep brain stimulation, and even watched video footage of some of the live surgeries. Some doctors claim that this technique can make their Parkinson's patients feel much better and lessen the amount of medication they have to take.

The way it works is this. The surgeon drills two holes in the patient's head and inserts two wires inside while the patient is numb but awake. Then he moves the wires around and asks the patient for feedback, until he finds the exact position in the brain where the tremors and dyskinesias originate. After a recuperation period from the surgery, the patient comes back to have the two wires attached to a pacemaker, which is inserted just under the patient's skin. When necessary, the settings on this pacemaker can be adjusted with minor surgery, just like those on a cardiac pacemaker.

After reading up on all of this, I attended a Parkinson's support group at the Robert Wood Johnson Hospital in New Brunswick, about a 45-minute drive from my home. I was the youngest person there. Only one other person was using a walker, and he was seventy. Two of the men in the group had had DBS and were feeling much better. My hopes soared.

I could hardly wait for my next appointment with Dr. Fahn.

"Dr. Fahn, I've been reading up on DBS surgery," I began. "Do you think I could benefit from that procedure?" I held my breath.

His answer came back without the slightest hesitation. "I'm sorry, Mrs. Reinman. Because of your dizziness and balance problems, you would not be a candidate for DBS."

Poof! My bubble burst.

Old and New Friendships

My sister's grandson was getting married in Rockland County, New York, and I would have loved to go to the wedding. For my sister, it was the first wedding of a grandchild, and she had only one sister with whom she could share her joy. Me! I wanted so much to be there for her, but it was not realistic. I didn't think I could tolerate the two-hour drive from my home. And besides, the reception hall was three flights up and not handicap accessible. I stayed home and felt bad for my sister. And for me.

A short while later, one of her grandsons in Eretz Yisrael was engaged to be married. The wedding would, of course, be in Eretz Yisrael. That one was out of the question. If I couldn't make it to Rockland County, how could I even think about going to Eretz Yisrael? I had come to terms with it. There were some things I could do and numerous things I could not do. I accepted it. But that didn't mean that I was happy about it.

The scope of my life had shrunk. A pattern had begun to form that has lasted to this day in one form or another. I spent many hours of the day in my workroom, with my computer, a daybed and various mementos of my accomplishments from my years as a teacher. I sat in my chair, the power recliner I had inherited from Bobby Ima, with pillows behind my back and my head and another supporting my right arm. Sometimes, I had practically no conversation with friends, even if they had walked all the way from the other side of Lakewood on a Shabbos afternoon.

I found it easier when two friends came together. I'd listen to them talk and just kept quiet. Ironically, I had had such a powerful voice as a youngster in the choir that I was sometimes told just to move my lips to avoid drowning out the other singers. Well, things had certainly changed. My voice didn't drown out anything anymore.

My family and friends would try to arrange a steady flow of visitors for me. Everyone wanted to help. Bayla Stein called my daughter and said, "Devora, give me a job. What can I do?"

Devora took her up on her offer. "Bayla, it's difficult for me to put people on the spot and ask them to visit. After all, I'm the daughter, and people would feel uncomfortable saying no to me. And sometimes it happens that a few people come all at once, while at other times no one comes. Would you be able to be in charge of her visitors? That way, people can be honest about what they can and cannot do."

And so, a unique group was formed among my family, friends and neighbors. It is almost like a club dedicated to helping me but having a wonderful time doing it. We have Chanukah parties and other events together. On Tishah B'Av, we all gathered in my house to watch the videos that others were watching elsewhere.

My visitors began taking two-hour slots each week to keep me company and to help me with whatever I wanted to do that day. They expanded my little world and filled it with smiling faces and loving voices. I am more grateful to them than I can say.

As my condition deteriorated, I was surprised and touched by the way many of my friends, old and new, came through for me and still do. Bayla has become a pro at filling up the days according to how I am feeling and what I can handle. She talks to me constantly about the schedule and what is or isn't working. And of course, she takes her own slot Tuesday mornings when she comes with Debbie Friedman. All three of us have so much fun. It's amazing that visiting the sick can be such a blast. Ophra Charnas comes every week, spends a lot of time with me and sometimes takes me out for a ride just to enjoy the fresh air and the scenery. My old friends Liba Friedman and Yehudis Mueller come together one night every week. Batsheva's best friend Hennie Halpert, who is like our adopted granddaughter and calls us Bobby and Zeidy, comes often just by herself, and we have a wonderful time together; her mother, Naomi, my daughter's next-door neighbor and close friend, also visits me regularly. My daughter's other next-door neighbor, Fraidy Rokeach, sends me delicious fish for Shabbos. Her husband's grandmother, Zeppy Rokeach, and my mother were best friends.

Some of my friends' children, many of whom I've known since they were babies, also visit me regularly. I love them dearly and have a great time with them, but I wouldn't exactly call them my friends. Bracha Malka Indik is the exception. The Indiks, Dovid and Feigi, are our next-door neighbors and close friends. During the good times, we joined them on Shabbos, for the Friday night *seudah*, many times. As it became more difficult for me to walk, they often came to us and brought their food so that the burden should not fall on my caregivers.

Over the years, I became very close with their daughters Elisheva and Bracha Malka. I taught them computers and spent many hours with them doing all sorts of graphics projects. My bond with Bracha Malka was especially strong. When she went to seminary in Eretz Yisrael she called me at least once a week without fail, and ever since she came back, she practically lives in my house. Despite the difference in our ages, I consider her among my closest friends. When we expanded and renovated our home, we made a large dining room, and it was always in my mind that I wanted to use that dining room to host a *sheva berachos* for Bracha Malka. If I could live to do that it would make me very happy.

My ability to have so many visitors without them tripping over each other I owe to Bayla Stein. She is a gift in my life. We were friends when we taught together in Ilan, but now she has become like a sister to me. Because of her, people can assist me without compromising my dignity. Because of her, my friends are there for me spiritually, davening and reciting *Tehillim* on my behalf, and they're here for me practically as well. I never thought I would be the kind of person who feels lonely. But the harder it becomes to join in conversations, the quieter it gets and the lonelier I feel.

These visits have become the focus of my life, not only because they keep me occupied, but also because of the deep friendships they have produced, friendships that have enriched my life more than I possibly could have imagined. Some of these were old friendships that had sort of gone into dormancy but blossomed again under these new conditions. In fact, they've become much deeper than ever before.

One of these friends was Frieda Schreiber. We were schoolgirl friends who kept up with each other because we both lived in Lakewood after we were married. We attended each other's family *simachos* and saw each other once in a while, but our lives did not really intersect. But I guess old friendships never die. They just doze off. Under my new circumstances, Frieda once again became one of my staunchest friends, always there to spend time with me and take me wherever I needed to go.

And then there were the new friendships. Rivky Kleiman, whose mother is a friend of my sister, started coming to see me regularly. Once she brought a friend, Yocheved Galy, who also lives in Lakewood but whom I had never met. Yocheved and I really hit it off, and she has been coming to visit me just about every week ever since.

I've also developed new and interesting friendships with Osnas Weitman, Malka Danziger and Rivkie Kanarek, all of whom I've known for many years without being particularly close. A few years ago, Yossel wrote a commentary on the Torah called *Abir Yosef*. Osnas started coming over and learning it with me. The pieces were very familiar, because I had heard many of them at our Shabbos table, but I enjoyed hearing them all over again. When Osnas couldn't come, Malka and sometimes Rivkie came and learned it with me. Yossel could not get over it. He says that he knows of no other author whose wife studies his work every week. He is very honored and pleased. That makes me happy, too.

Very often, some of the grandchildren come on a Friday night to eat with us and keep me company. The girls stay with me. The boys go to shul with Yossel, and Devora arranges for a neighbor to keep us company until the men come home. We have the meal first, and I try to make time to play a game or two until they go home.

On Shabbos mornings, I get up early because my friend Avigayil Brailofsky comes at 9:45. I need the time to get dressed and eat breakfast before she comes. She lives less than a half-mile from our home and walks over rain or shine to come and daven with me. She says all the *tefillos* out loud in the tunes that were popular in our youth, and I listen. I try to sing along, and I argue with her about the tunes; she uses a different one for every *tefillah*. We have a lot of fun together. I wish I could still sing. Shabbos day, Devora or Chaim usually come for the *seudah* with their families, and Idy Yoffe, who lives about a mile away, comes afterward and spends the rest of Shabbos with me.

Other friends, Goldie Schechter, Chumie Meisels, Nechamie Miller and Miriam Kahan, helped me write this book. When I could no longer type on the computer, I'd dictate to them. One of them kept interrupting with her own thoughts, constantly trying to guess what I would say next and ending my sentences for me. "Hey, am I writing this book, or are you?" I asked. We laughed a lot and had a great time.

When my friends come, we usually play a game called Upwords. It's similar to Scrabble, but all the letters have the same value and you score points by piling words on top of each other, reaching ever higher. The game is sort of a metaphor for my life. Even in my declining condition, I am still trying to rise, to ascend, to better myself, to lift my spirits and the spirits of those around me in my own small way.

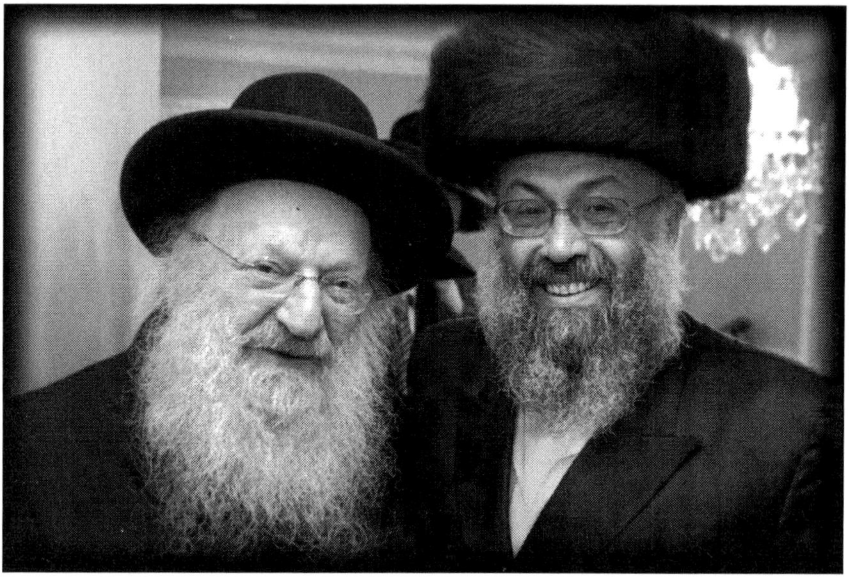

The author's husband and Rav Mattisyahu Salomon at their *siyyum* on *Mesechte Arachin* on Shushan Purim in the author's home

The title of this book, *Upwards*, is a play on words on this game, which has become such an important part of my life. It also reminds me that I should never despair and always strive for growth. I once heard that if Hashem puts you on your back it means that He wants you to look upwards. I can relate to that. I'm trying.

Although I play the game with many of my friends, Bayla is my stiffest competition; she knows the dictionary by heart. But I beat her once in a while, and all in all, I am a pretty good player.

During these last few years, I've also been playing Upwords weekly with Rebbetzin Miriam Salomon. Her husband, Rabbi Mattisyahu Salomon, had come from England to become the Mashgiach of the Lakewood Yeshivah. He and Yossel have been learning together for fifteen years and are close friends.

When they first began learning together, I met the Rebbetzin at a party and introduced myself as the wife of her husband's *chavrusa*, study partner. The next time I met her she couldn't remember who I was. "I'm so sorry," she said. "I'm meeting so many new people, and it's hard for me to remember everyone's name."

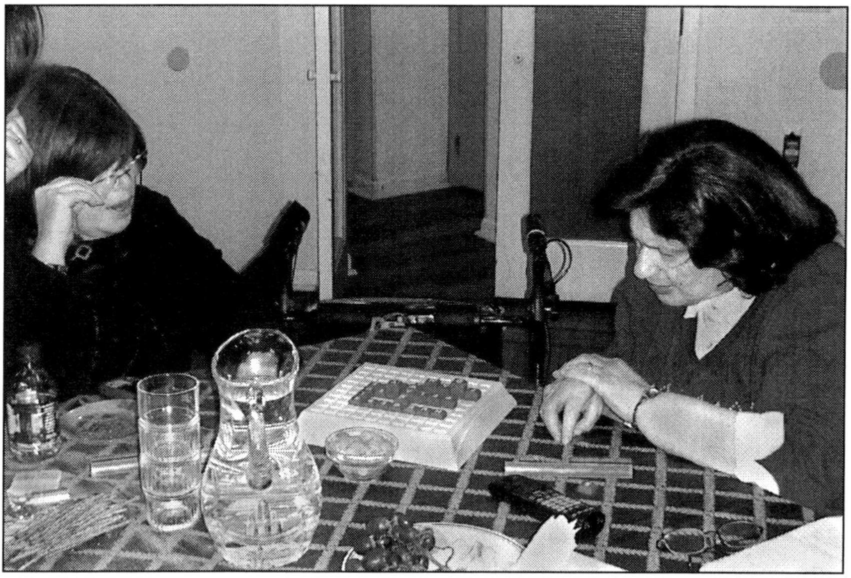

The author playing Upwords with Rebbetzin Salomon

"Well, you'll be seeing me again. I'm the wife of your husband's *chavrusa*."

The next time we met, her eyes lit up. "You're Shami Reinman," she said.

I was in the Salomon home a little while after that, and Rabbi Salomon said to me with a twinkle in his eye, "My wife remembers who you are."

Several years ago, the Rebbetzin suffered a heart attack. She had a procedure done in Columbia Presbyterian and then went to recuperate in Leisure Chateau, a nursing home in Lakewood. I visited her when she came home and brought an Upwords with me. Ever since then, we've been playing every Wednesday, either in her house or in mine . We set out cookies, dried fruit and drinks, and we have ourselves a little party. My friend Frieda picks her up and brings her to me or vice versa. Frieda joins us in the games. Rabbi Salomon told Yossel that he is very pleased with this arrangement as we are both in need of *chizuk*, emotional support, and we are providing it to each other. We have become very close over the years, and the Wednesday games have become one of the highlights of my week.

As my talking became more difficult and less understandable, I sought out other games we could play if my friends tired of Upwords. We played Russian dominoes, Rummikub, Overturn and Uno, among others.

Even now that I can barely move the Upwords tiles with my shaky hands, I can still beat most of my friends at it. The games keep me busy, and they keep me sharp. I play to keep myself occupied, to stay relevant, to interact with my friends. I play to stay alive.

One-Sided Conversations

Extrovert that I am, friends and games were still just part of the picture. The center of my life had always been my home and my family, especially my husband. As time went by, things were becoming strained between Yossel and me. He didn't quite know how to deal with me in my situation, and I wasn't sure what to do about it either.

Feeling helpless, I continued to distract myself. I spent time researching my illness, enjoying my children and grandchildren, visiting with friends, learning things to elevate myself spiritually, and running to new doctors. One day, I made an appointment to see a Dr. Golbe in Robert Wood Johnson Hospital in New Brunswick.

Yossel was nice and took me there, even though he wasn't quite sure why I was going to another doctor if I did not intend to leave Dr. Fahn. Both of us knew I was grasping at straws.

"How can I explain it to you?" I said. "I just want to hear another doctor's opinion. Do I have MSA or Parkinson's? Should I take more medicine or change what I'm already taking? Will he understand what I mean when I say that I feel dizzy? Should I go for genetic testing? Are my kids at risk? If he helps me with even one medication, it's worth my time going down there."

We arrived late, but the doctor had waited for us. Whew! I was so relieved. I handed him my emergency card with all my information typed out. Meds I was on, vitamins I was taking, surgeries I'd had in the past and so forth. He was very impressed.

Then I handed him the list of my symptoms. I think he was impressed with the work I'd done, but he barely glanced at it. Dr. Golbe put me through a series of tests to see what I was capable of doing. Some of the tests were familiar to me from Dr. Fahn's office; others were new. I didn't get perfect scores, but I didn't fail the tests, either.

I'm sorry to say that this new doctor was no more helpful than any of the others.

Meanwhile, now that I was no longer working and had to have full-time help at home, money had become tight. Yossel was trying to come up with creative solutions to the cash-flow problem. Our financial situation made for some stressful moments, and that was on top of the emotional stress that had moved into our home after I was diagnosed with Parkinson's.

I'd always stood by my husband. I was very proud of all his accomplishments in learning and his writings, his commentaries and his other books. I always introduced myself as Yaakov Yosef Reinman's wife. I'd sold my engagement ring so that he would be able to publish his writings.

We brought up four children, and we did a pretty good job judging by how they've turned out. We'd always enjoyed each other's companionship while traveling together. We'd taken trips to Eretz Yisrael many times, to France, Belgium, England, Italy, Spain, Venezuela and many places inside the United States.

Our house was always vibrant and alive, full of friends and family. As a teacher, I've had many students visit our home over the years, and it never took long for the ice to be broken with my husband. The conversations were fun, as we challenged each other and our guests with riddles and opinions.

Yossel is funny, witty and very personable. He loves arguing his point — to death! He believes in his political views, and he makes sure everyone around him knows what they are. And he is very persuasive at bringing others around to his point of view. In other words, communication is his strong point. But it was getting harder and harder for us to communicate with each other. My conversations with my husband were usually one-sided. He did most of the talking, because it had become so hard for me to say anything. And when I did speak, he often couldn't grasp what I was saying. He'd lean toward me and say, "What? What? I don't understand you," until I finally made myself understood.

Yossel didn't like it when I was too demanding. I was grateful to him because he always did so much for me — shopping, taking care of my medications and always running to the pharmacy when I needed something. He just didn't like it that every time I saw him, I had something for him to do. I didn't like it much, either. But there wasn't much else now. Now that we really couldn't communicate normally, I guess I was trying to keep up the relationship by asking him to do things for me. And that wasn't really working. After a vibrant shared existence, we had begun to lead essentially separate lives. And that made me sad.

I tried to see things through my husband's eyes. I really did. I imagined what it must be like for him to lose the energetic, extroverted wife he'd married, who for so many years had been his companion and best friend. In her place there was now a sick and dependent woman who needed help with everything, who could hardly make herself heard, who spent her days attended by aides and helpful friends.

I love and respect my husband, and I know that he still loves me. But I also know that he is slowly being crushed by his own sense of loss.

Back when I was first diagnosed with Parkinson's, Yossel and I were poring over some literature about the disease. The brochure offered some instructions for the caregiver.

"The caregiver," I said, "that's you."

Yossel shook his head. "I'm not a caregiver," he said, and he was right. He doesn't have the temperament or the patience to be a caregiver. He never had the patience to feed our children when they were little or to look through a technical manual when he got stuck. I understood that I couldn't expect him to be something that he wasn't, but I was sad that our relationship had to suffer because I couldn't keep up with him any longer.

A few times a day, I could hear him come upstairs from his office to the kitchen to get a drink, and I'd hear him exchange a few words with Sadie before he went back down to his office. Sometimes, they'd laugh. I couldn't help feeling a pang of jealousy. Over supper, he would have long and interesting conversations with Shulem, and every once in a while, he'd make an effort to involve me, but it didn't really work.

Where was I headed? If I felt so isolated now, how would I feel in the future when I would probably have to spend the rest of my life in a wheelchair?

It was depressing.

A Time for Joy

The dizziness came back stronger than ever. After all my efforts to find a solution failed, the doctors and therapists concluded that it was being caused by my disease. There was no solution.

That evening, I just sat by the table and cried my eyes out. Yossel felt so bad for me. He tried his best to console me.

"I'm so proud of you, Shami," he said. "I'm amazed at how well you're handling everything that's happening to you. It's really incredible."

I really appreciated his sympathy, but I knew that I just had to move on and learn to live with it.

We'd married off our three older children years before. Now it was time to step into the world of *shidduchim* again. Shulem, our youngest son, was ready to search for a marriage partner. He had met a few *shidduch* suggestions, but so far nothing had panned out.

And then there was Brochie Stern, daughter of Yeshaya and Rochel Leah Stern, from Boro Park; good family, smart, funny, beautiful and so sweet. The *shidduch* took off from the start. Shulem probably would have proposed to her after a few dates if he thought she would accept. But he wasn't sure, so he didn't.

But as it progressed, Shulem wanted to bring her home to meet his parents. Of course, that was the proper thing to do, but how would I manage it? Would I be able to talk coherently? Would my shoulders spasm? What would she think of me? And would it affect how she felt about Shulem?

I needn't have worried. She was everything we expected and more. I wasn't the life of the party, and I said as little as possible. But nothing happened to undermine my dignity. I just sat there listening to Yossel converse with her very easily, and I was happy. When they got to talking about languages, she recited the Four Questions of the Seder in speedy French. Yossel, who speaks six languages, got a kick out of that.

After numerous meetings over the course of several months, Shulem and Brochie were engaged in February 2010. Traditionally, the deal is officially sealed by drinking a *lechaim* together in the home of the prospective bride. The Sterns lived in Boro Park, and that was where we were going to be the next evening.

Well, wouldn't you know it? A big snowstorm blew in that night. Snow was falling in heavy waves, and a gusting wind was pushing it into huge white drifts. Suddenly, I heard a popping noise, and all the lights went out. It was pitch black in the house.

I told my husband that I'd heard something pop. He didn't believe me.

"Nothing happened," he said. "It's just a regular blackout. They'll fix it soon."

But I knew that I'd heard something. And then I smelled a burning odor. The house was on fire! Though I couldn't see any flames, I knew we had to get out of the house immediately.

The smell was coming from my computer room downstairs, and when Yossel smelled it, he immediately called the fire department. He thought there might be an electrical fire in the wall of the computer room. Yossel told the fire department that his wife was a Parkinson's patient, and they promised to come immediately. And they did.

Devora and Sadie helped me plow through the snow banks to a neighbor across the street, while Yossel waited for the fire trucks in front of the house. As I watched from my neighbor's window, I saw the red fire trucks coming down the block. When they reached our driveway, they discovered the trouble immediately. A fallen branch had snapped a wire near our house. The smell in the computer room was coming from a line filter that had burned through. *Baruch Hashem*, no damage had been done.

Well, back to reality. It was time to get dressed and head to Brooklyn for the *lechaim*. Devora and Sadie helped me back across the street. The downed wire was lying loose in the driveway, and the snow was very deep. I tried my best, but it was just too much for me. I just sat down in the snow and laughed. Yossel finally created a path for me with his feet and helped me into the house.

I had to get dressed by candlelight, because the power was off on the whole block. Luckily, there was still some hot water in the water heater, and we were able to shower normally. Finally, we were ready to leave, and I wondered if I could come back to a dark and cold house. Where would I go to spend the night?

But first things first. I would worry about where to sleep after the *lechaim*. Brochie's parents were very gracious. Her mother did her best to make me comfortable and keep me involved. She settled me into a chair in the living room where the ceremonial *lechaim* would take place. Five minutes later, however, the crowd sort of moved over to the kitchen, and I was stuck in the living room alone. So I asked my granddaughter Blimi to help me, and we made our way to the kitchen. And wouldn't you know it, by the time I got there and took a seat, everyone was ready to return to the dining room for the *lechaim*. So I struggled back to the other room to join them.

The rest of the evening passed in a blur of good wishes and cries of "*Mazel tov!*" I was truly happy for my son. We had been blessed. At eleven o'clock, one of my neighbors called to inform us that the power was back. Whew! That was a relief. At least, I could go home to my own bed.

And now it was time to think about the wedding. Yossel and I had discussed where my book should end, and we both agreed that Shulem's wedding would be a good place to do it. I hadn't believed I would survive to escort my son down to the *chuppah*, but now it looked as if I would actually be part of it in the living flesh. The book would then end on a high note, an emotional moment, a small triumph over the disease.

I had many things on my mind as I prepared for the wedding. I was busy with the regular things like clothing and makeup. We had to make sure there was a comfortable couch on which I could rest during the wedding and a good rolling office chair that I could use instead of a wheelchair. But this wedding held a special ordeal for me.

Although I could barely walk, I was confident I could escort Shulem down to the *chuppah*, supported by him on one side and by Devora walking next to me on the other side. The problem would arise once we got to the *chuppah*. Before the *kallah* takes her place beside the *chassan*, she circles him seven times, escorted by both of their mothers. Would I be able to manage those seven circuits under the *chuppah* in my condition? Should I even make the attempt?

We talked it over with Rabbi Salomon, and he suggested that I do only one circuit and then sit down. Everyone would understand.

Shulem had been unaware of the discussions until we raised it one night at supper.

"I don't understand, Ma," he said. "Ma, why can't you go around seven times?"

"Mommy could trip and lose her balance," Yossel told him. "Or she could get dizzy and fall. That would be worse than not going around the full seven times. Once is more than enough."

I tried to say something, but I'd lost the power to project my voice. I raised my hand to get their attention and said, "I'll see how I feel at the time."

As the wedding drew closer, I was busy with my needs. The arrangements usually made by a groom's mother were undertaken by others. Brochie's mother chose the flowers, and Yossel paid for them. Yossel hired the photographer and videographer. Chaim took care of the band. They tried to involve me, but it was just for form. I felt left out.

When the wedding day, June 14, 2010, finally arrived, I was nervous but ready to face whatever came. The day of my dreams and prayers was here. Yossel and I were walking our youngest child down to the *chuppah*. The band played a soft, moving melody as Devora walked down the aisle next to me. She held the candle in her left hand and supported me with her right.

The enormity of the moment gave me an extra charge of energy, and I decided then and there that I would do the full seven circuits. And I did. Then I sat down on a chair that had been prepared for me under the *chuppah*. My husband gave me an approving look that said, "I knew you'd pull it off!"

I spent the rest of the wedding in a rolling armchair with wheels. I danced with my friends and family from my sitting position. They held my hands, and I sensed their love and heartfelt blessings. It was an evening filled to the brim with joy.

Caregivers and Companions

My need for assistance grew as time passed. At first, all I needed was a full-time housekeeper who could also do some personal things for me when they were too difficult for me to manage on my own. But as time went on, the focus shifted from housekeeping to Shami-keeping. I needed help with everything — getting dressed, taking a shower, going to the bathroom, getting ready for bed at night.

Sadie had been with us for two years during the earlier stages of my disease. When she left, the agency sent us Miriam Escobar, an older woman from El Salvador. She had worked for Rabbi Elya Ber Wachtfogel and his family in South Fallsburg, New York, taking care of his mother-in-law until she passed away in August 2010. Miriam was a very fine and caring woman, but the work was a bit much for her. She had little patience for children and worked hard to keep everything sparkling clean and tidy. She spoke hardly any English, so Yossel spoke to her in

Spanish. She used to write her shopping lists in Spanish. Yossel liked that, because he learned the Spanish words for celery, mushrooms, garlic, eggplant and many other foods and household items.

Unfortunately, Miriam's daughter back in El Salvador was battling breast cancer at the time, and Miriam was terribly worried. She flew back to El Salvador when her daughter had surgery. Rabbi Wachtfogel and my husband paid for her ticket. When she finally left in March 2012, Elba from Peru took her place.

Because my disease had progressed by the time Elba arrived, her job called for her to be with me seven days a week. She was also paid almost twice as much as Miriam, which had already been quite a bit of money. The financial pressure on Yossel was mounting, and I could see it taking its toll.

Elba's English was a little better than Miriam's but not by very much, and Yossel got more opportunities to practice his Spanish.

Elba was, to put it bluntly, a difficult woman. Although she took good care of me, she was controlling to the point of being emotionally abusive. For example, she refused to let me have my laptop in bed. She often didn't answer when I called for her. If I asked for a toothpick, she would say I didn't need one so that she wouldn't have to go get it. In June of that year, Yossel was invited to be scholar-in-residence in Manhattan Beach, and we were put up in the home of a family that was away for Shabbos. Elba went shopping in the afternoon and didn't come back for hours. Yossel was furious.

When we had guests, she would refuse to cook for our guests.

"I just cook regular," she'd say.

"Yes, regular," Yossel would answer, "but for three more people."

For some reason, she was afraid of Yossel, who is not very scary, and she always gave in. If I complained to Yossel about something and he brought it up with her, she would get upset with me for telling on her.

Yossel kept asking me if I wanted to fire her. I was reluctant to say yes, because who knew what her replacement would be like? At least Elba took care of my physical and sanitary needs. I hesitated to start over with someone new who could be even worse.

"It's up to you," Yossel said again and again. "You pull the trigger, and I'll fire her."

Finally, in August 2012, I pulled the trigger. Yossel fired Elba. But before he did that, he interviewed her replacement. The interview took place in my daughter's house without Elba's knowledge.

He'd called the agency, and they told him that they'd be sending down three people. Sarah was due to meet Yossel in the morning, Victoria in the afternoon and a third woman the next day. Sarah, the morning appointment, never showed up for her interview. Yossel met with Victoria, the second young woman, in Devora's house. The interview went well. So well that he canceled the third candidate and hired Victoria on the spot. She stayed in my daughter's house while Yossel went home to fire Elba. She told him that she was not surprised, that a message from Heaven had informed her that she was about to be fired. Yossel gave her half an hour to pack her things, then sent her off to Queens in a cab.

Victoria Buenaventura is a young Mexican woman in her early thirties. She owns a shop in Cuernavaca, Mexico, but an economic downturn made her decide to come to the States to earn some money. She told Yossel that she had experience taking care of an older patient and provided a reference. Yossel was so impressed with her that he didn't bother to call the reference. It wasn't until some time later that she confessed that the reference had actually been a friend of hers who'd agreed to play the part of a former employer. Victoria had never taken care of a patient or a household before, but she really needed the job and was confident she could do it well. We forgave her for the deception, because it turns out she was right. We could not have asked for a more wonderful caregiver, and she's still with us today.

Victoria is patient, intelligent and extremely caring. We are like soul mates. We even share the same birthday. We talk and laugh together, and I really enjoy her company. She often knows what I'm going to say even before I say it. She tells me about her life, and I tell her about mine. Now and then, we play canasta. I would play Upwords with her, but her English, while pretty good, is not yet good enough.

Victoria is a free spirit who just loves adventure. She gets antsy just sitting at home inside the four walls. Fortunately, she drives, and we go out together a lot. We go shopping for hours and hours. We go down to the beach. We go out for pizza or ice cream. Sometimes, Yossel comes along and we go out to lunch in a local restaurant. Victoria is more than just a great caregiver. She's become a close friend.

Trips and Hurricanes

My body kept on betraying me in new ways. It was now an everyday occurrence for me to send messages to my legs and find that they simply refused to listen. Victoria would tell me to move to the right or the left, but my legs would not respond. I was getting stiffer and stiffer. In the mornings, my arms were very stiff, too, though they tended to loosen up as the day went on.

It was also getting harder for me to eat and drink. I was slowly losing my ability to eat and swallow. I cannot say that this surprised me, because it is so common with neurological diseases. I just never thought it would happen to me. But there it was. There was no denying it. Would I need to have a feeding tube implanted in my stomach or was I going to die first?

Thoughts of death only made me want to embrace life more tightly. In December 2012, my husband went to Eretz Yisrael to visit our Israeli grandchildren, who missed us very much. My going along was out of the question. If we somehow did organize the trip so that I could come along it would be such a huge, complicated and expensive operation that Yossel would probably just cancel the whole thing and stay home. So he went by himself.

Well, not quite. He took our granddaughter Blimi with him for company. They planned to stop over in Venice on the way home. That didn't bother me so much, since I had once been to Venice on an Ilan school trip. Before they left, Yossel and Blimi practiced speaking Italian so that they would be able to make themselves understood when they got there. Yossel had done the same years earlier when we went to Rome for a few days. He managed to communicate in Italian, but the only word I knew was *andiamo*, let's go. I had to say that a lot when he spoke to people in Italian. After we came home, he basically forgot his Italian, but now he was refreshing his skills together with Blimi.

So while these two were away having fun in Eretz Yisrael and Italy, I decided that I would go away, too. I would fly down to Florida. Batsheva and Hennie, her friend, had a few days off from work, and they offered to take me to a hotel in Miami Beach for the weekend. Then, on Monday, I'd move into a friend's house in Boca Raton, and some of my friends would meet me there. My parents used to go to Florida every year for at least a few weeks without taking us along, and ever since, I've had this thing about going to Florida. I think it was like forbidden fruit that I was finally allowed to taste.

When I looked more closely into the matter, however, I discovered that the house in Boca was bare. There was only a table, four folding chairs and beds. There were no handicap facilities or comfortable couches. Although it was very nice of them to let me have the place, I knew it wasn't meant to be, and I canceled the trip. I'd made reservations to go to Florida the year before, and then I had also backed out. The tickets were nonrefundable, and we lost the money. It was a good thing I hadn't made reservations again and lost even more money this year.

When my husband came home from Eretz Yisrael and saw my disappointment at not having been able to go to Florida, he came through for me and said that we would go together. I was so pleased.

The trip was not exactly like the dream vacations we'd enjoyed on our earlier trips to Florida. I missed those days. This time, we took rooms at the Marco Polo in Sunny Isles. We stayed there for nine days, including Purim.

It was not an easy experience. In fact, it was very taxing. I don't know why it surprised me, but all my aches and pains had snuck into my baggage and come with us. We rented a van, but I couldn't climb into it. So I had to stand on a pot we borrowed from the hotel. We went to eat out a lot, and I felt that everyone was staring at me in my wheelchair. I saw a woman imitating the way my mouth twitches. Sometimes, I drooled, and Victoria was always instantly there with a tissue. I felt very self-conscious.

But there was also a lot of good. The weather was beautiful. We had rooms overlooking the ocean, and I would sit on the terrace every morning for a long time. We went to cafes and restaurants. We also went to Bayside a few times. Purim was on Sunday. For Shabbos and Purim, we went to our friends the Marlowes in North Miami Beach, and we attended a party in their neighborhood. Some of my students from Bais Kaila were there as well, and they were very sweet to me. The best part of the trip was that I got to spend a lot of good time with Yossel.

The author davening on the porch in Florida

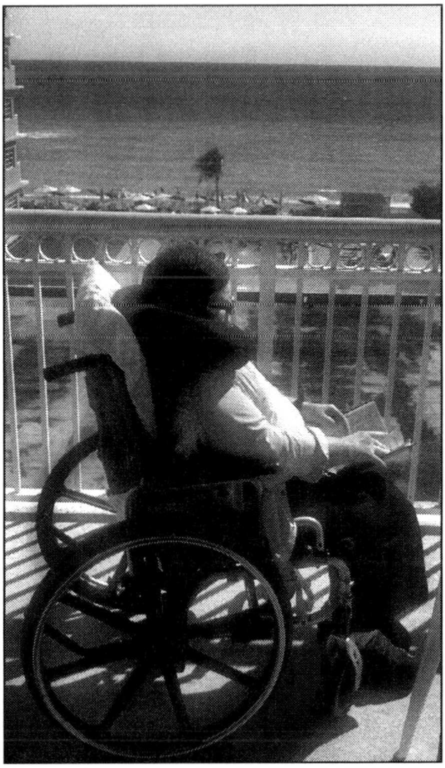

A few days after we returned from Florida, I was changing into pajamas in the bathroom when I slipped and almost fell. All that kept me from hitting the floor was my right hand's grip on a handicap bar. I called for help. Victoria came running, but she wasn't strong enough to lift me back into a standing position all by herself.

"Grab onto the bar with your other hand as well," she said. "I'm going to get help."

She came back two minutes later with Tzipporah Lapa, my neighbor and dear friend, also not a very big and strong person. I was hanging on for dear life. I knew that if I let go I could hurt myself, maybe even break something. Tzipporah held one of my arms and Victoria the other, and together, they managed to stand me up.

After Victoria got me into bed, I tried to calm down, but I couldn't. I felt more helpless than ever. I couldn't even go to the bathroom without constant supervision.

Thankfully, Victoria brought a positive attitude to everything we did. She encouraged me to walk, always coaxing me just a little past my comfort zone. Her pleasant personality made it seem like fun, like an adventure.

But as much as Victoria had become part of our lives, she also had a life and family of her own. When she had to return to Mexico to be with her mother for a week, she found us a Colombian woman named Fabiola to take her place. Fabiola spoke decent English and was quite nice. She always ran from task to task. She wasn't used to walking.

Fabiola was in and out of our lives for some time. In fact, she was with us when Superstorm Sandy struck a day after Victoria had returned from a vacation. Fabiola was still with us, and she remained with us until life returned to normal, which was well more than a week. The rain poured and the wind howled. And then the lights went out. I was terrified. I didn't know how long we would be without power; it didn't seem like it would come on again anytime soon. What was I to do without light or heat or hot water? Would trees fall and come crashing down on our house?

Volunteers from a local aid organization put a gasoline-powered generator outside the house and ran many extension cords into the house through the deck door. Our floors were like a web of wires leading to the refrigerator, lamps, space heaters and my hospital bed. The volunteers also had to return every six hours to refuel the generators.

The days went by. Some parts of Lakewood had power restored, but not our block. It seemed that a transformer had blown and they were having a hard time repairing it. Eventually, it was repaired by a crew from Alabama. It was dangerous for me to remain in the house with all those wires and generators. Also, Shabbos was approaching. Could we stay in the house under those conditions? We had to find other options.

Rabbi Moshe Peretz Schwartz, the rav of our shul, offered us the use of a small bungalow he had set up on the shul grounds for the occasional guest who needed to be close by. The bungalow had a kosher kitchen, a dining room, two bedrooms and an office with a couch. Best of all, the power was on! We accepted gratefully. Victoria and Fabiola ran back and forth from the house bringing food from the fridge and freezer and any other things we would need.

We stayed there for about a week. After we came home, there was an unexpected snowstorm. Oh no, I thought, here we go again. But the snowstorm didn't do much damage. The power stayed on, and we stayed home.

Sometimes, that's what life feels like. It's just one thing after another!

It Ends When It Ends

My book was drawing to an end. I had written most of the material and dictated the rest to my friends. We had thought that the happy climax of my book would be Shulem's wedding, if I lived that long. But I was still alive, and more milestones had appeared in my life. One year after their wedding, Shulem and Brochie had a beautiful little boy. Surely, this belonged in the book. Okay, so the book would end with the birth of my youngest son's first son, unless something else happened that would make for a nice ending.

Yossel suggested that the book should end with the book's completion. It ends when it ends. That's not as crazy as it sounds. A big part of my book is the process and the experience of putting it together. Sending off the book to a publisher would make a fitting conclusion.

There was only one problem. Yossel had promised that after I finished the book he would edit the manuscript and rewrite those parts that needed rewriting. Besides being a great writer, he is also an experienced editor of hundreds of books. In the past, he'd rewritten books by well-known personalities, such as Rabbi Mattisyahu Salomon, Rabbi Shlomo Freifeld, Rabbi Yissachar Frand and Rabbi Boruch Eliyahu Goldschmidt, simulating their voices through the text. Who could be more qualified to work on my book? But it wasn't happening. He was finding the task much harder than he'd expected.

He kept trying and trying, but he was getting exactly nowhere.

"I sit down at my desk," he would say, "fully intending to work on your manuscript. But I find myself doing other things. I have a real block when it comes to this book."

When I asked him how the book was coming along, he would say, "Please don't ask me about it. It just puts more pressure on me and makes it even harder. I know you're waiting for it, and I'm doing my best to get it done."

So I stopped asking him outright, but the unspoken question was there all the time.

"Stop looking at me that way," he would say. "That's just like asking me. I'm trying. I'm trying."

I understood that the block was an emotional one. This was just too hard for him. The story of my life and my illness was not something he could approach in a detached, objective way. It hurt too much.

Finally, we reached a compromise. We'd find someone else to rework the manuscript for me, and Yossel would polish it. Unfortunately, the person we found produced work that didn't sound like me! We were back at square one.

Then I had an idea. We'd just sold the house I'd inherited from my father, and we had some cash on hand. Of course, we would need every penny for the mounting expenses of my care. We already had full-time help seven days a week. Who could predict what I would need in the future? And what would we do when the money ran out? But in the meantime, we had a little money in the bank.

I handed my husband a hefty check. "I'm hiring you," I said. "Maybe getting paid will help break through your writer's block!"

It helped a little. He did manage to rewrite the first few chapters, but then he got stuck again. He was going crazy. He had made me a promise, and he always kept his word. He'd made a commitment to me. He had even been paid! But he simply could not do the rewrite. What was even worse, he couldn't write anything else, either. When he sat down to work on another of his books, he felt guilty that he wasn't working on mine. And when he sat down to work on mine, he wasn't getting anywhere. It reached the point where he dreaded being in the same room with me, because he could sense the weight of the question I wasn't asking.

Finally, I decided to let him off the hook. Did I have a choice?

"Don't do the book," I told him. "It's killing you."

I remember the look of relief and guilt that filled his face. We talked it over, and I told him that he needed to find someone else who could do the job instead of him. We agreed on one name. Libby Lazewnik.

Libby is a well-known author in Orthodox Jewish circles. She's written many books for adults and young-adults, and I've always enjoyed her writing. It was Yossel's job to track her down and offer her the job. He finally located Libby in Baltimore, and called her one night. She agreed to come up to Lakewood to see us one day that summer.

It was a good meeting. I was impressed with Libby. She listened with sympathy and asked pertinent questions. When she left, Yossel and I were both hopeful that we'd found the right person to shape my writings into a book. From that point, we were sure, Yossel would be able to take the book to its final stage. He knows better than anyone else what kind of words and expressions I would use and the type of things I would say, and he knows my life better than anyone else. I understood that it was too emotional and complicated for him to put together and rewrite the book, but once a book was patched together from all my manuscripts, notes, revisions and dictations, even if it had many rough edges, he could work his editorial magic on it. He's done it for so many other people. Now he would do it for me.

Meanwhile, my life was continuing to unfold, and there was plenty to keep me busy and interested. Chanukah was coming, and I wanted to throw a party for all the dear friends and family who'd given me so much love and support, but it was more than I could handle. My friend Suri Kaszirer, whom I have known since childhood and who comes to visit me every Monday night, very kindly offered to arrange the party and have it in her home.

The party took place on the fourth night of Chanukah 2012. I came early, because I didn't want everyone to see that I needed to be supported on both sides just to get across the room. About fifty women came, including Rebbetzin Salomon. My daughter-in-law Brochie showed up with Dovi, my adorable grandson; everyone enjoyed watching him crawl to me calling "Bobby! Bobby!" before scooting back to his mother.

Avigayil Brailofsky spoke first. She was very funny as she described her experiences davening with me on Shabbos morning, and the songs we sing. Everybody was laughing. Then she spoke about her froglike singing voice, and everyone called out for her to sing something. So she sang a song that she'd composed for when her children fought with each other. As soon as she starts singing, her children stop fighting with each other and unite to make her stop. We laughed until we cried.

Gittie Ryback spoke about how all the rocks fought to be the pillow for Yaakov's head until they all turned into one. And that is what happened with the wonderful group that had formed around me. They have become close friends, unified in their love for me, who come to visit more for themselves than for me. I was so moved. I realized that I was part of something bigger that was happening, part of a bigger plan.

After the speeches, we played a game that Bayla and Debbie had made up. It was a lot of fun. The game involved reminiscences about old Lakewood. The topics covered banks, stores starting with an S, anagrams and old stores like Wexelbaum's and Estherdale. It was very well done, and everyone had a good time.

The party was wonderful. I went home in a haze of golden memories. Old and new.

The School Dinner

One evening, Rabbi Yisrael Schenkolewsky and Rabbi Shmuel Mayer, my former principals at Bais Kaila High School, came over to our house to meet with my husband. They asked him if we'd be the guests of honor at the upcoming 2013 Bais Kaila annual dinner.

Yossel accepted, because he didn't really have much of a choice. Our granddaughters are students in that school, and we simply could not refuse to help. I agreed that we had to accept, but I insisted that Yossel go while I stayed home. I wanted to stay out of the public eye as much as I could. In the end, Yossel convinced me to go to the dinner with him. He said that many people would be coming just for me, and I had an obligation to be there.

Memories came flooding back from my years at Bais Kaila, where I'd been a successful and popular teacher for ten years. I'd had some interesting run-ins with Rabbi Schenkolewsky, some of which we still laugh about. For instance, when I needed him to fix something in the computer lab, I was such a persistent nudge that he stopped taking my calls. But that didn't deter me. Instead of calling from home or the school, I'd go over to Rabbi Schenkolewsky's downstairs neighbor and call from there.

Once, I called him at school and told the secretary I was his mother.

A minute later, he got on the phone. "Hi, Ma."

"It's Mrs. Reinman," I replied.

He was fuming. "Don't you ever do that to me again. What do you need?"

Another time, I arranged for someone from the fire department to come down to the school and address the entire student body about safety measures. The speech took place in the gym. Unfortunately, I didn't know that there was no regulation CO2 detector in the gym. Rabbi Schenkolewsky and Rabbi Mayer were sure they were going to be hit with a $25,000 fine for that missing CO detector.

Rabbi Schenkolewsky called me. "Who gave you permission to use the gym?"

Meanwhile, we were all holding our breath to see if a fine would be imposed.

The next day, the fire commissioner drove up in a red car and handed Rabbi Mayer an envelope. Rabbi Mayer opened it with trembling hands, fully expecting a hefty fine. Instead, he found some dot-to-dot books and coloring books, and a note saying, "Please give this to Mrs. Reinman for her students." All had ended well, but Rabbi Schenkolewsky was still pretty exasperated with me!

There were many more memories, mostly about the girls, with many of whom I'd formed lifelong relationships. Those were some very good times, and now it was time to show my appreciation by coming to the dinner and greeting all the people that would be coming in my honor.

I couldn't believe how many people had come for me. So many colleagues, friends and family from Lakewood, Brooklyn and beyond. So many former Bais Kaila students, some of them grandmothers already! So many former Ilan students. So many of the people I loved had come out for me, and it touched me to the bottom of my heart.

As I looked through the dinner journal, I saw that many of my friends and family had placed ads in our honor. As I read them again and again, I was warmed by the fond memories they brought to mind. My very good friends Gittie Ryback and Leah Trenk, who were my former principal and assistant principal at Ilan, wrote about my days at Ilan. I was glad to see how much they had appreciated my work during those wonderful years.

In honor of our dear friend and teacher

Mrs. Shami Reinman

To work with Shami is to love her!

During her years as a teacher in Ilan, there was never a job too menial or too monumental for Shami. Though the computer room was her primary domain at Ilan High School, her influence reached everywhere and touched everyone. Whether it was printing the *Kolenu* newsletter, publishing the yearbook, chaperoning school trips, graduation trips, Bais Yaakov Conventions or hosting Shabbat meals at her home, Shami was always available.

Shami is a master at making work fun. No matter what Shami is dealing with, laughter is an essential part of the program. It was no wonder that we used to spend hours chasing students — and teachers — out of the computer room and into the classes they were supposed to be attending! Shami's wit highlighted her wisdom.

After decades of teaching — and reaching so many students — Shami had the art of teaching down to two basic principles. Love every student and never underestimate the power of humor and a warm smile.

She taught her students volumes by example.

She is still teaching all of us volumes by example.

We love you, Shami!

Mrs. Gittie Ryback Mrs. Leah Trenk

My dear friend Bayla Stein wrote about my facing life with joy. That doesn't mean that I'm not suffering every single day, every single minute. But I'm still happy to be alive, happy to be with my friends and family, happy to be able to laugh together and have fun. So I guess it is true that there is a lot of joy in my life.

> Dearest Shami,
>
> On this occasion, I want to acknowledge the gift that you have given to me and all your friends who know and love you. I want to thank you for your joy which you share with all of us. Our visits are punctuated with giggles and laughs, funny observations and fond memories. We are all attracted to your *simchas hachaim,* which shines forth in all situations.
>
> I will never forget last Purim. I came to bring you *mishloach manos* with my children. Shami, you were sitting in your large armchair dressed up as Savta Simchah. You had on a big floppy hat, with a bird perched on its brim. You had a large black bag packed with little *tchatchkes* for the children. Each person that came into your room that Purim received a gift for life. They got to see you, dear Shami, a vestige of your former self, yet an enthroned queen, a *savta* full of *simchah.*
>
> The Ribono Shel Olam has given you many talents and *kochos.* I thank you for sharing your *simchah* with all of us.
>
> Bayla Stein

I'd dreaded being in the spotlight at the dinner, but it turned out to be a very enjoyable evening, though I'd never admit it!

Two Letters

Just recently, I received two beautiful letters sent to me for inclusion in the book. They express certain things about my life and my experiences that I could not express myself. The first letter is from my friend Avigayil Brailofsky, who comes to daven with me every Shabbos morning. I mentioned earlier that she does this, but I couldn't even begin to describe the wonderful experience of our davening together. She does.

Dear Shami,

Every Shabbos morning has a special feeling for me. I open my front door and walk down Buckwald Court. Whether its glittery snow, orange leaves or springy air, I enjoy this quiet stroll alone to Steven Lane. I knock and open the door. I like the way your house smells; something like Murphy oil and a woodsy scent.

"Is Shami ready?" I ask Victoria.

"Yes!" she says as she wheels you into the kitchen.

"Gut Shabbos, Shami!" I greet you.

This Shabbos you are all dressed up with your sheitel and jewelry.

I take out your special Siddur, the one you inherited from your Bobby Ima. We sit at the round dinette table with the sun streaming in from the window behind you.

I've learned that the *Shechinah* rests above the head of a person who's sick, so I'm glad I'm facing you. We exchange small talk, and I make sure your pillows are arranged in all the right spots and your tissue box is handy.

"Ready?"

You nod, and I begin. We start with *Modeh Ani* and move into the *berachos*. We say *Asher Yatzar*, using the familiar chant we used back in our elementary school days.

I look at you mouthing the words. You seem expressionless. It's hard for me to see you like this. I know you since our Bais Kaila High School teaching days, where your verve and spirit left an unforgettable impression on me. But I know you're still there, and this is just part of the disease.

Sometimes I catch a glimpse of your feelings. I was so shaken up when I davened with you on Rosh Hashanah in Kimball Hospital. Tears were running down your cheeks; it was the first time I ever saw you cry. You told Devoiry and me, "I feel bad I didn't always say *Asher Yatzar* with enough thanks."

We continue with melodious *Elokai Neshamah*. I think about how your soul is peeking out more as your body shows up less.

After *Matir Assurim* you say, "That's me! A prisoner in my own body."

We move on to your absolutely favorite part. *Ranenu Tzaddikim*. You are very connected to this *tefillah*, and no matter how late we start you will not skip it; I think it has something to do with your grandmother's attachment to it. We sing it to the old "*Ivdu es Hashem*" marching tune.

We begin *Baruch She'amar* with a rousing, "*Hareini* ..." After that it's *Mizmor Shir*. Whether it's Pirchei and the Rabbis Sons (your era), or Miami Boys Choir, MBD, Avraham Fried (my era), you favor the oldies. You especially enjoy "*Mikolos mayim rabbim* ..." and in *Yehi Chivod* two more golden oldies: Rumrumrum .... and *Rabbos Machshovos*. At these times, I can see you back in camp singing your heart out.

We chant *Ashrei* to the traditional school tune, and now we reach the challenge: the five *Hallelukahs*. You want a different melody for each one. You've prepared the tunes during the week (with Goldie Schechter) and penciled them into your Siddur. I try my best to fit your choice to the words, but inevitably I end up squishing some verses into the song with an off-tune *kneitch*, and we both burst into laughter. It's also funny when we try to add a seasonal touch to davening. Like Pesach time when we did *Az Yashir* to *Dayeinu*! I really can't get your grandfather's three-part *niggun Echad Yachid* right, and you patiently put up with my missed beats each time. This past Shabbos you almost choked from laughter from my mangled tune. I really should prepare like you.

When we first began our davening together I would suggest the *hartzige* slow stuff that I thought would be nice. Isn't davening supposed to be emotional? But you insisted on fast joyous melodies, and it's been a very emotional experience. Happiness is an emotion too! The only tear-jerker you allow is *Nishmas*. You selected the wistful "Sefer Torah Niggun" ("I was made way back in 1843 ...") for this *tefillah*, and at the high part the harmonies flow through your lips. The words are touching, "*Ki chol peh* ... therefore every mouth shall offer thanks to You, and every tongue shall vow allegiance to You ... every knee shall bend to You and every spine shall prostrate itself before You." And then we sing this verse high, "*Kol atzmosai*, all my bones shall say ... who is like You? ... we shall praise and glorify You!

"*Borchi nafshi* ... bless Hashem, O my soul, and let my innermost being bless His holy Name!"

But what's if not? What's if a mouth can hardly express itself? What's if a knee and spine don't respond? How can someone bless Hashem?

Shami, you are the answer.

I've had Shabbosim where I heard echoes of your beautiful voice and some weeks that it was faint, but you don't stop. When you turn the page of your Siddur I feel that Hashem views it as hands outspread like eagles. And when you strain to sing it's like your mouth is as full of song as the sea.

Once while we were singing *Avinu Av Harachaman,* which tells how Hashem is so compassionate, I looked at you as the twins were sitting on each side of you caressing your arms. I always think about how you are ensconced in such a lovely home with loving family and oodles of friends around you. You are beloved by so many. And it's obvious Hashem loves you so much.

We get one more chance to say *Ranenu Tzaddikim.* And then we sing *Yishtabach* with enthusiasm. We have a different tune for every one of the paragraphs after the *berachah* of *Yotzer Ohr.* Carlebach compositions go with almost everything. And finally we're up to *Shema.*

You are able to cover your eyes and focus on Hashem. I marvel at you. Would I be able to daven if I were in your situation? Would I be able to ignore the pain and discomfort week after week and daven for an hour and a half?

One Shabbos I woke up feeling achy. I wanted to lie in bed all morning. But then I thought of you, and I dragged myself to your house. If you can do it, how could I not?

I've learned that the structure of our prayers parallels the architecture of the *Beis HaMikdash.* I feel like I've been walking through with you and now we are about to enter the *Kodesh Kodashim.*

I walk to the corner, and you daven in your chair.

I don't take it for granted anymore that I can stand and bow during the *Amidah.*

But although you're sitting in your wheelchair I have a feeling you are in the innermost chamber with Hashem.

The men are home by now. We kiss *gut Shabbos* and I leave.

I'm different from when I arrived.

They say davening changes a person. Davening with you, Shami, has changed my life.

As I walk down Cedar Row, I think about the fourth *Hallelukah*. We sing it to a tune that's very close to your heart. "Shir, shir, I'll sing to Hashem, lalalalala as long as I live."

That's you, Shami. You're singing to Hashem as long as you live.

And I'm learning how to sing from you.

Avigayil

I was very touched by her letter, and even though she exaggerates, the picture she draws of our time together is so true. I love it.

The second letter is from my daughter, Devora. I am privileged to have wonderful children, and I think there is a place in this memoir for my daughter to express her love for her mother. I cherish every word.

Dearest Mommy,

If we said anything unusually nice or helpful when we were young, you'd always say: "Can I have that in writing?" Recently, I have realized that, although we always tell you we love you and very much mean it, it may seem a bit of a throwaway statement, like "see you later" or "have a good week."

And now you are putting out a book about your journey. I have been struggling with the decision of whether I would like to contribute a few words to your story and try to express how much you mean to us all; indeed, to put it in writing. Can I capture my thoughts? Do I want to say them? I do, but it is harder than I thought.

How can we explain just how much you mean to us all? And how could you understand the overwhelming attachment I feel toward you?

You have battled with so many things over the course of your life and always with grace and joy. Now you are battling the effects of a terrible illness, yet you have never given up. I can't imagine you ever will.

Mommy, you are a great woman. You don't act as though you know it. You have an endless, wide-eyed curiosity about life. You delight over a new game or a child's performance. Your faith is so simple that it is the greatest faith I have ever witnessed. R' Mattisyahu [Salomon] once told us that holiness is something that must be experienced; it is difficult to teach. Mommy, you are a holy woman. And I cry as I write this, but you deserve to hear it. Your joy in performing mitzvos is amazing. Your *minhagim* are your anchor. You get excited to come to the Shabbos table even if you are in pain.

Through your life you have worked tirelessly to provide for us, support Totty in his learning and writing and give us your love every chance or way that you knew how. You joined me in every decision I made and cheered me on. When I switched gears, there you were, cheering me on! You continue to be an inspiration for bringing up my own children, and I see a lot of your kindness and empathy in them.

Mommy, your acceptance of all people warms me. Your mission has always been to make everyone you meet into a friend. You have always been that way. I think you got that from your mother. If someone had a personality quirk that irked you, you would find a way to love them and make them into a friend. It is not that you were immune to people's character defects or negativity, you just worked on finding a way to like them. You don't give up on people. Ever. And your friends, my friends, Cindy's friends, Batsheva and Blimi's friends and the list goes on – they are now your life-long friends.

There is no particular age group that you associate with. So much so, that Chanala and Raizy, my adorable nine-year-old twins, come visit and bring along neighbors on Shabbos. They're all coming to play with Bobby Reinman.

It does not stop. When Shmuel had a Purim party in our house for the *bachurim* in his *shiur,* I saw one of his friends talking with you and crying over your pain. Because everyone loves you. Mommy! Everyone, because people know that they are important to you.

When Shmuel was engaged to Gayil [see Chapter 49], they were on the boardwalk, and they saw a stuffed pillow that had the word love embroidered on it. Shmuel's first reaction was "Let's play that game. I want to win that pillow for my grandmother." It took a lot of tries, but Shmuel did win it and proudly brought it to you, just like he so excitedly brought his *kallah,* Gayil, to meet you. Of course, you enveloped her with love. You personify love to the children. Berel, who's a big *bachur* already, feels as though you are lost when he does not stop in. He makes it his business to visit and call. You make each and every one of your grandchildren feel so treasured. There is always enough attention to go around.

The physical loss you've been suffering so early in your life didn't make you change your path. It just gave you opportunities to find creative solutions to still live fully. You are an avid researcher and naturally inquisitive. You find ways to keep updated by reading a variety of subjects from home. Vast numbers of books still adorn your shelves, as reading has been another lifelong passion. Sadly, because of deteriorating eyesight, books can no longer bring you the same joy they once did, although you allow me the pleasure of reading to you when you are well enough. Not to be deterred, though, you plow through audiotapes and phone *shiurim* when alone to help ease the monotony of endless days in bed.

What I really hope you can understand, with all this burbling, is that I could not have wished for a better mother, and feel incredibly lucky that we remain so close, emotionally and geographically.

You have only ever supported me, and rarely criticized. My children have had a wonderful role model right on their doorstep, one they admire and respect. They have learned the importance of family and can see how you go on working determinedly to put everyone first, despite your failing health. In their eyes, too, you can do no wrong.

You really are the most giving and exceptional person I've ever met, and I'm blessed that you are my mother.

Everyone loves you, but no one could possibly love you as much as I do.

Devoiry

What can I say? I am blessed.

Seeking Answers

My neurologist was fairly certain that I had MSA, but I needed to know for sure. I wanted closure. On my next appointment, I brought up the subject again. Again, he told me that MSA was indicated because the progression was too fast for classic Parkinson's. Nonetheless, he suggested that I take a SPECT brain DaTscan, which might give us some indication.

We made an appointment to take the test at Columbia Presbyterian, and I went there with Victoria and my friend Chaiky Schreiber, Frieda's daughter-in-law. DaTscan is an imaging technology that uses small amounts of a radioactive drug to help determine how much dopamine is available in a person's brain. I was handed a horrible drink that burned my throat. Chaiky sat next to me and cheered me on.

The first scan was not conclusive, and the technician had me come back in the afternoon for another scan. Unfortunately, the second one was also inconclusive. All I'd wanted was some clarity, but it seemed that it was not to be.

The next few weeks passed with no new insights or milestones. I watched winter turn gradually into a new spring. On a sweet morning in early April, I made an entry in my almost-finished manuscript, which I'd been using more and more as a kind of diary to record the impressions, thoughts and feelings that filled my days.

> April 4, 2013
>
> Yesterday was my Hebrew birthday. I am 63. My body is slowly deteriorating. I cannot stand unless you want a hug. I have trouble swallowing liquids, and therefore, it's difficult to impossible for me to take my pills. I take them with yogurt or applesauce and that makes it easier. At night, I try to get it down by chewing an orange. It takes about an hour. My body is forgetting how to chew and swallow.
>
> I do not know what is going to happen. I tried to get answers, but I am left with questions. I gave it all I had, trying to learn my diagnosis so I can be prepared for what will happen to me. Will my end come quickly, or will it be torturously slow? Will my younger grandchildren remember me at all? Will my older grandchildren remember my sick self or my real self? Will they recall how I drooled and they offered me tissues? Or how much fun I used to have with them?
>
> All the answers will come as they happen, I guess. For now, I try to be as happy as I can. I try not to complain or be unpleasant.
>
> What the end will be, only Hashem knows. I accept whatever He sends my way, though of course I am fearful. I am grateful for every day that I have, and I'll take it as it comes.

The Final Journey

Originally, we had planned to end the book with the momentous milestone of the marriage of Shulem, our youngest son. But time had brought more milestones, although not on the same magnitude, and the question of how to end the book still remained somewhat open. As I said before, Yossel had suggested that it end when it ends, and I agreed. But still, it would have been nice to finish on a high note, a climactic event in my life besides the completion of my book.

And then it happened. Shocker of shockers, Shmuel Follman, Devora and Tzvi's son, my oldest grandchild, was engaged to be married. I was beside myself with joy. A married grandchild! Who would have believed I'd live to see that?

The girl was Avigail Greenes from Los Angeles. One year earlier, her family had moved to Eretz Yisrael, but she remained to go to school in Brooklyn. Most of her family was here in the United States, but technically, she lived in Eretz Yisrael. So

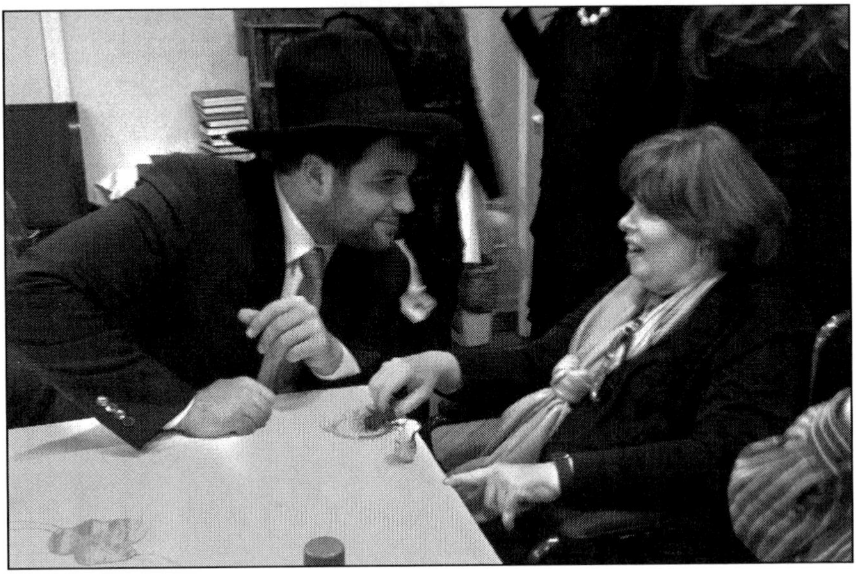

The author with her grandson, Shmuel Follman,
at the *lechaim* in the Salomon home

where would the wedding take place? I was hoping desperately that it would take place here so that I could attend. Yossel and I both knew that a trip to Eretz Yisrael in my condition was out of the question.

Ultimately, Avigail's parents decided to make the wedding in Eretz Yisrael, and that was the end of that. In the back of my mind, I thought that maybe I could indeed pull off a trip to Eretz Yisrael, but I didn't even mention the thought to Yossel. He had been around the block before with my trips canceled at the last moment. He could not handle any more of my fits and starts. But the image of my beloved grandson's wedding halfway across the world wouldn't leave me, and I did speak to my children about it.

By this time, Victoria was part of the family, and she would have offered her opinion about what could and could not be done. Yossel had a lot of confidence in her, especially after she had made the Florida trip work so well. But Victoria was back in Mexico when the engagement was announced; her sister had come to take her place during her absence.

One day, without telling me about it, Yossel called Dr. Lebowitz from the car so that he would have perfect privacy. "I have a question," he said. "Our grandson is getting married in Eretz Yisrael, and I know that she desperately wants to go. Do you think she's capable of making the trip?"

"Yes, she can," said Dr. Lebowitz, somewhat to Yossel's surprise. "With the proper arrangements and support, she could do it."

With the doctor's consent, Yossel decided that he would try to make it happen. I was nearing the end of my life, and I should not be deprived of this fantastic joy if it was at all possible. Still in his car, he called his travel agent and asked if Victoria, who has a Mexican passport, would need to apply for a visa to visit Eretz Yisrael. The travel agent assured him that Mexico was on the list of countries that required no visa for Eretz Yisrael. The major hurdles had been cleared. With doctor's permission and Victoria's assistance, the trip to Eretz Yisrael was suddenly a possibility.

He put away his phone and headed home to see if I wanted to make the trip. He didn't know what I would say. Of course, he knew that I wanted to go, but was I ready to undertake the heavy strains of such a journey?

He came home about a half-hour after Victoria returned from Mexico. When he saw her, he said, "Welcome back, Victoria. Did you hear the news? Our grandson is engaged, and the wedding is in Eretz Yisrael."

"I know," she replied. "Your wife told me. And she wants to go."

"Hmm," he said, and he was just about to come see me when the phone rang. It was Shulem.

"So, I was thinking about the wedding," Shulem said.

"Yes?" Yossel asked.

"Um ... maybe Mommy should go?"

"Hmm. Interesting idea."

No sooner had he hung up the phone when it rang again. This time it was Chaim. Apparently, he had also been thinking that I should go to the wedding.

Yossel burst out laughing. He knows me very well, and he could see my hand maneuvering behind the scenes.

Finally, he confronted me directly. "So, it seems you're thinking that you'd like to go to Eretz Yisrael for the wedding."

I didn't deny it.

"Who'd you tell about it?"

"Just the kids."

"And what about your friends?"

"Oh, my friends ... yes."

"Which ones did you tell?"

I had the grace to blush. "Actually ... all of them."

So the decision was made. We were going. Yossel purchased business-class tickets so that I'd have a more comfortable trip, booked rooms with handicapped accessible bathrooms in the Ramada Renaissance Hotel in Jerusalem, and reserved a rental car. The numerous other arrangements were left to Victoria, who was a marvel. Nothing fazed her! She always had the same, calm answer, "It'll be okay. Don't worry."

A few months earlier, my son Berel had come to visit me from Eretz Yisrael. Victoria had seen a video online about the custom of placing brief notes containing prayers into the Western Wall. She had also discovered that King Solomon had prayed that non-Jews, as guests in the House of Hashem, should get positive responses even more quickly than Jews. So Victoria asked Berel to take a *kvittel* from her and place it into the Wall when he went home. She spent a long time writing it in Spanish. Then she folded it into a tiny square, sealed it with scotch tape and gave it to Berel.

Now, as we planned feverishly for our trip, she confided to us that one of the prayers on her *kvittel* had been answered. She'd asked Hashem for a chance to go to Eretz Yisrael.

I was thrilled to be making this trip, though I knew that it would take a supreme effort on my part. Things that other people take for granted had become an ordeal for me. The slightest mishap could set me back in disastrous ways. It would put a burden on my family, too. But I put all such thoughts out of my mind and focused on the incredible joy of seeing my grandson getting married.

The wedding was set for Tuesday, June 11, 2013, in the hotel where we were staying. It had originally been booked in a different hotel, but at the last minute, it had been switched to the Ramada Renaissance. What a great stroke of luck for me! Now I wouldn't have to get into and out of cars to get to the wedding. I could just go down the elevator from my room in my wheelchair and be there.

We decided to come to Eretz Yisrael the week before the wedding to give ourselves a chance to rest and recover from our journey. We were scheduled to leave for home on the Thursday after the wedding, arrive in New Jersey at the crack of dawn, and spend Shabbos at home resting.

As it turned out, we didn't end up doing much resting in Eretz Yisrael. Victoria was thrilled to be in the Holy Land for the very first time, and she wanted to see everything. On Thursday and Friday, we went to the Kosel, where I poured out my heart in prayer. I'd been davening to Hashem constantly since I'd been diagnosed, but there was a special feeling as I stood at that Wall. I knew He was listening to me and loving me. He'd given me this illness for a reason. He'd bestowed this trip to Eretz Yisrael on me as an incredible gift. As I murmured words of *Tehillim*, I absorbed the holiness of the place and felt it continue to envelop me as I was wheeled away.

That same day, we visited Berel, Sora Rachel and the children. Have I mentioned how much delight I take in my grandchildren? I love being a mother, and being a grandmother is even better. Boruch, Malkie, Ezriel, Dovid, Aryeh Leib and Levi Yitzchak are totally adorable. The baby, Elimelech, is a pudgy little bundle of joy, always laughing and emptying the cabinets in their kitchen. The youngest, Raizy, wasn't born yet. On Shabbos, we invited them to come to the hotel for the meals, which was a rare and wonderful treat for the children. Victoria, being a good Catholic, took advantage of the time to tour the sites that were special to her in the Old City.

On Sunday, we headed out into the country with Victoria at the wheel; she wanted to drive and get to know the country. I sat next to her, and Yossel relaxed in the second seat. Our first destination was Tiberias, an ancient city on the Sea of Galilee.

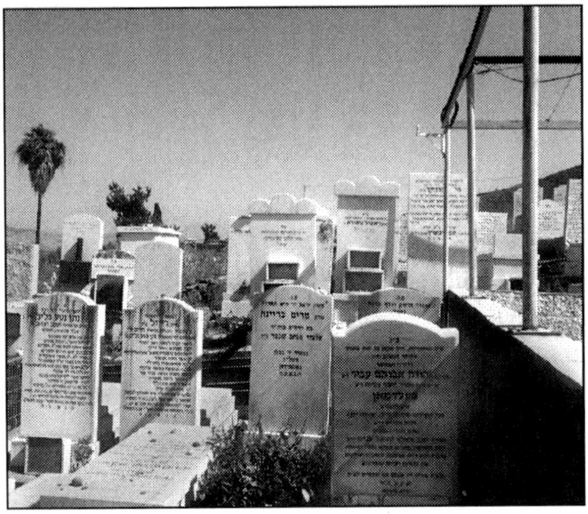
Bobby Ima's *kever*

My grandfather and grandmother are buried there. We drove there alongside the Jordan River. On the roadside, we saw a camel, and of course, Victoria had to take a ride and get pictures.

The cemetery in Tiberias is old, crowded and on a hillside. It was a struggle to get up the hill, but I wanted desperately to daven at my grandmother's grave. Yossel dragged me up the rocky path in my wheelchair until we reached Bobby Ima's headstone. I shed a few tears and offered up some *tefillos*. I didn't think I would ever return to full health, but I davened to Hashem, in the merit of my great and holy grandmother, that I shouldn't suffer so much and that I should at least enjoy the time I have left to me. Bobby Ima was always such a symbol of strength. I davened for some of that strength to sustain me now.

From Tiberias we headed to Netanya, all the way on the other side of the country on the Mediterranean coast. On the way, we detoured so that Victoria could visit other places of interest to her. Nazareth is an Arab city and looks like one. As was to be expected, Yossel had friendly conversations with some of the people we met. At no time did we feel we were in any danger. In Netanya, we took a long walk on the gorgeous boardwalk, and we had dinner in a restaurant on the beach while we watched the sun sink into the blue sea. Then it was back to Jerusalem.

On Monday, we visited the Kosel again . Our son Chaim arrived that day together with Louie Follman, my son-in-law's brother. Shulem arrived a little later. Chaim and Louie joined us, and we set out for Tel Aviv, where we hoped to see the Mitzpeh observation deck. Unfortunately, Louie's state of the art GPS took us to a small house on a back street. We had a good laugh and headed for the famous Tel Aviv beach. We walked along the boardwalk for a long time, everyone taking turns pushing my wheelchair. We passed two Oriental women in motionless stances. Yossel said they belonged to a Chinese quasi-religion. We stood next to them and took pictures. We passed a few Arab women in head scarves. Victoria wanted to take pictures with them, but they refused.

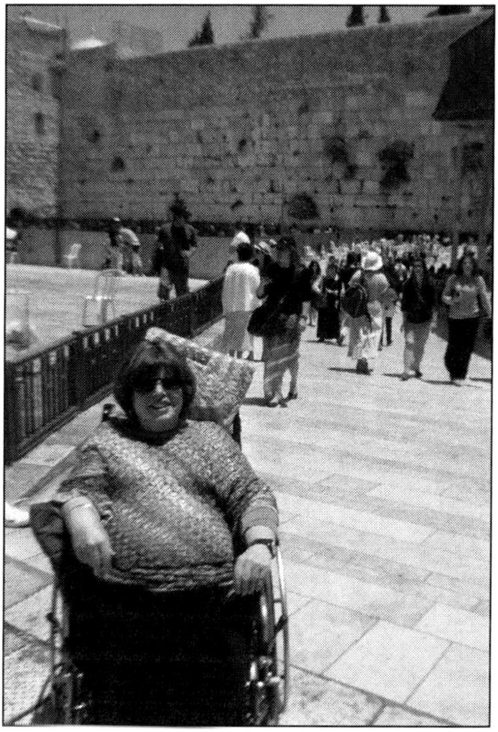

The author at the Kosel

From the beach in Tel Aviv, you can see the picturesque old city of Jaffa, and that is where we headed next. It was getting dark and windy, and I stayed in the car while the others went to the boardwalk. A group of about six or seven Arab women in hijabs and headscarves stood talking on the boardwalk nearby. Yossel asked Victoria if she wanted a picture with them, and having been rejected before, she told him not to bother. He asked them anyway, and they graciously agreed.

After Victoria got her pictures, Yossel got into a long conversation with them, while Chaim and Louie watched from the distance and smiled. The Arab women introduced themselves as Palestinians, teachers from Hebron. As a Jew, and a liberal-minded one, Yossel was fascinated by what they had to say about the burning issues in Eretz Yisrael and the Middle East. Yossel always likes a fresh perspective. He feels it gives him a much broader understanding of the issues. At the end, they invited him to visit their school in Hebron. That liberal he is not!

When he came back to the car, I said to him, “Why didn’t you bring them over? I’d have liked to be part of the conversation, too.”

“It would have broken the momentum,” he said. “I didn’t want them to stop.”

I understood perfectly well. That conversation would not have been possible with me participating. They would have stopped every few words and tried to figure out what I was trying to say. But I couldn’t help feeling sorry for myself, alone and out of things in the rental car. I had to content myself with hearing about the conversation from my husband afterward.

But there was too much going on to let me feel sorry for myself for long. Between sightseeing and davening at Eretz Yisrael’s holiest sites, every day was a whirlwind.

Finally, Tuesday arrived. Because it was too difficult for me to visit a hairdresser and a make-up artist, they came to the hotel instead. Everyone got ready in my room. It was like a huge party, with lots of laughter to punctuate the serious work of making

The author with her American children and grandchildren on Chanukah after the wedding

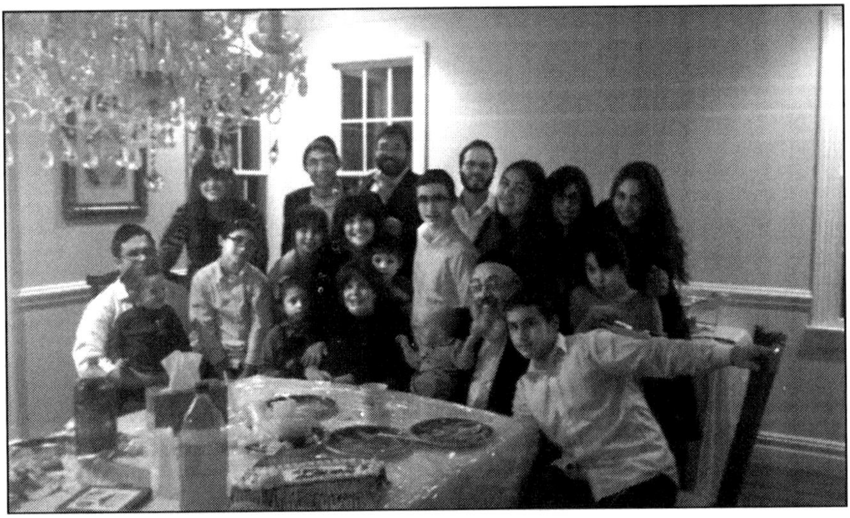

ourselves look presentable for the wedding. We were giddy with happiness and having the time of our lives!

By the time we were done, Devora and the girls looked gorgeous, and I looked pretty good, too. As I was wheeled out of the hotel to make our way to the outdoor *chuppah,* I found myself looking forward to the wedding with a special intensity. I'd already met my granddaughter-in-law-to-be, and we'd clicked immediately. I was eager to welcome that lovely girl into the family.

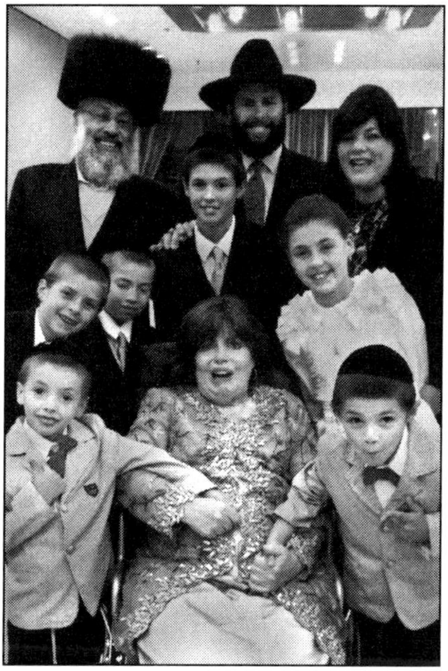

The author with her son Berel's family at the wedding

Even more than that, I was deeply aware of the privilege Hashem had given me to be alive and present at this wonderful event, surrounded by the people I loved most in the world. I watched as my daughter and son-in-law walked their son down to the *chuppah,* with a heart that was almost too full. Full of gratitude and happiness. And also filled with the nagging question: Will I live to see another grandchild get married?

The *chuppah* took place on the lawn, and the dinner was in the grand ballroom. Many of Shmuel's friends came, and the music and the dancing were rocking. I danced with the *kallah* from my wheelchair, gripping her hands tightly as we moved to the music. My pace was more sedate than it used to be in the past, but my heart was certainly whirling at full speed.

It was surreal. I couldn't believe that I had done this, that in my condition I had traveled all the way to Eretz Yisrael to share in this precious moment and that I had been able to travel all around the country and not just stay in the hotel. I felt intensely alive, and I was grateful for every moment of this joyous experience.

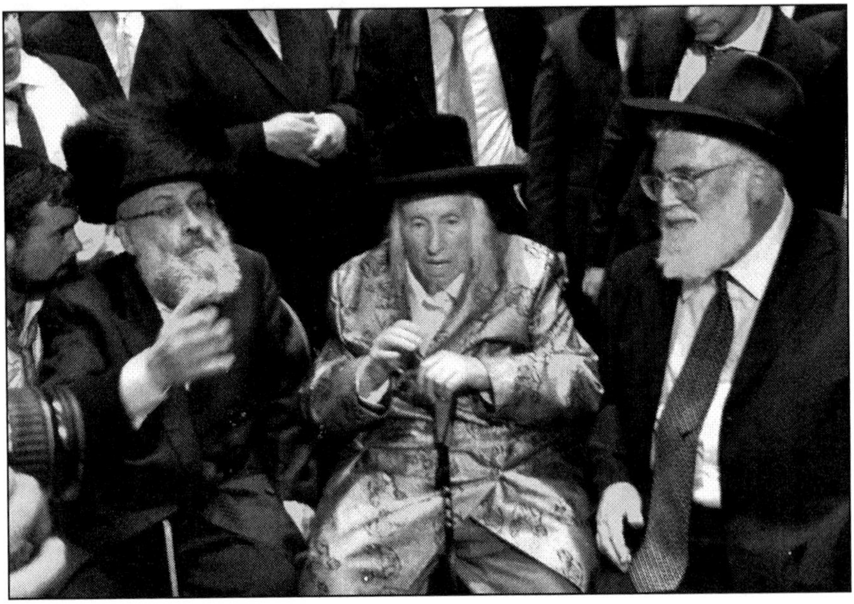

The Kalever Rebbe comes to the wedding

A big stir took place in the middle of the celebration when my great-uncle, the Kalever Rebbe, made an appearance. The Rebbe, now ninety years old, had once spent a Shabbos as a guest at our home in Lakewood, and he decided to show his gratitude by coming to give his blessings at the wedding. His arrival was a sensation . The boys crowded around him, singing in his honor and asking for his *berachos*. When things calmed down, the Rebbe sang *Solo Kakosh Ma*, a beautiful old song, and danced a *mitzvah tantz* with the *kallah*. On his way out, he had to push through a crowd of people begging for his *berachos*. His visit meant a lot to me, and even though it was a little bit of a distraction, I felt that it added an important dimension to the celebration.

On our last day in Eretz Yisrael, we started out with a visit to Kever Rachel. The place wasn't too crowded and the *kedushah* was in the air. I poured my heart out in prayer in the resting place of Rachel Imeinu, who certainly knew what it means to suffer. I davened for acceptance, for strength and for continued *nachas* from my family in the time I had left. Rachel's spirit had been unbreakable. I would try to be the same. I would try to never stop hoping, never stop clinging to life. To never stop seeing the parts of life that are happy and beautiful.

Afterward, we went to an ice cream shop called Waffle Bar in the Ramat Eshkol neighborhood. We had sinfully rich dishes and got chocolate all over ourselves. In the afternoon, we went to the Dead Sea. My granddaughter Batsheva came with us. We passed the camels again, and this time, Victoria, Batsheva and Yossel took turns riding the camels in the hot sun and having their pictures taken. Yossel was even wearing a *kaffiyeh* to lend him some local color! I, of course, watched all the fun from the car.

This time, though, my husband wanted to make sure I was part of things. He brought the camel over to the car to say hello to me. Lots of pictures were snapped. I appreciated his efforts. It seemed to be my lot now to be part of things, and yet not part of them. But it was better than nothing. A whole lot better!

Before we left for the airport, we went to a park in Ramat Shlomo, where we had a last picnic with Berel, Sora Rochel and the children. I played board games with the kids for a while, but the kids had too much energy to sit still; they wanted to run

With Berel in a park in Ramat Shlomo on the day of departure

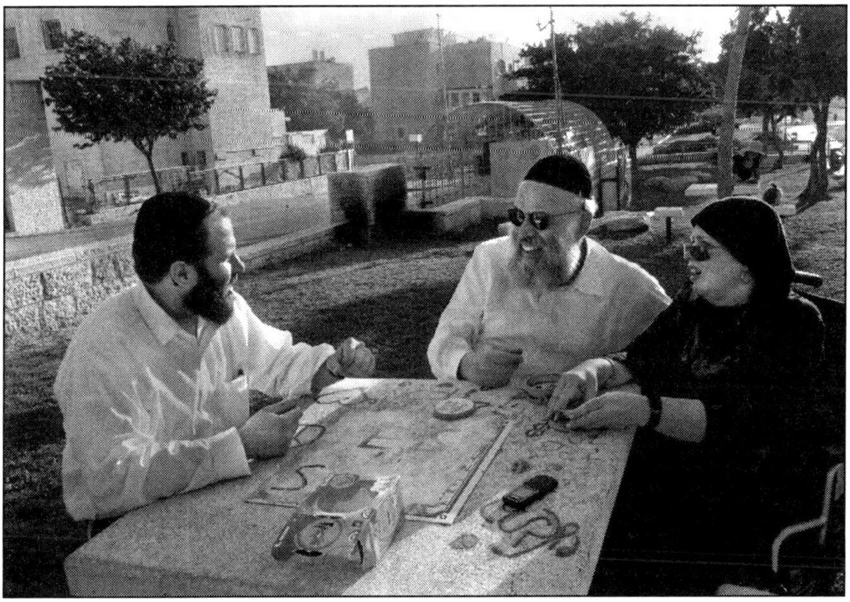

around and play soccer. One of my cute grandchildren felt bad that I couldn't join them. He looked at me and suggested sweetly, "Bobby, why don't you play by yourself for a while?" What a darling child! How I was going to miss him!

Then it was time for final hugs and kisses, trying to smile through my tears. It was so hard to leave my children and grandchildren behind. Each time we have to say good-bye, it's like ripping off a piece of my heart. Yossel wheeled me back to the car to pick up our bags at the hotel. It was time to start for the airport and the long flight home.

I gazed out the window for a last glimpse of Eretz Yisrael. My heart was full. It hadn't been an easy trip, physically, but I was glad that I had gone. I'd had the privilege of seeing my grandson married, another generation beginning to build a home and a family. I could have spent all my time in the hotel, but instead, I'd traveled the length and breadth of the land and poured out my *tefillos* into the holy air. I'd been warmed by the Mediterranean sun and by my grandchildren's smiles. I'd enjoyed a slice of real life on this trip, not invalid life, and it meant a lot to me. Life is a series of minutes in the here-and-now, and I felt I'd made the most of every one of them on this visit.

Now I was on my way home. I was looking forward to picking up my daily routines: the visits from my devoted friends, the learning, the games, the connecting. And in the background, every hour of every day, my love for my family.

In Lakewood or in Eretz Yisrael, I can only aim at being the very best person I can be. Wherever I go, I know I never travel alone. Now, more than ever, I have a sense that Hashem is my constant companion. He holds my hand and guides me, even in this frightening period of my life. He will never abandon me.

As we lifted off into the midnight sky, studded with millions of stars that have been there since the beginning of time, I remembered the words I'd written on my birthday.

> I accept whatever Hashem sends me, and I am grateful for every day that I have. I'll take it as it comes.

Acknowledgments

First and foremost, I humbly thank Hashem for granting me the privilege of writing this book. May it bring honor to His Name and comfort to His people. At this time, I want to thank my husband for encouraging me to write and for doing such a wonderful editing job after I was finished; special thanks to Libby Lazewnik and Judi Dick for helping shape my book into its final form. I also want to acknowledge the constant love and support of my family throughout this terrible ordeal. A special note of appreciation to my aides, Victoria Buenaventura and more recently Camila Lozano, for their tireless devotion, kindness and love; they are like angels sent from Heaven.

I want to express my deepest gratitude to all my old and new friends who found the time in their busy schedules to keep me company and brighten my days. I am listing your names in alphabetical order, because I do not want to give preference to one over the other. If I inadvertently omitted someone, please, please, please forgive me. I love you all.

Rebbetzin Miriam Salomon; Karen Aaron; Mary Abadi; Channy Abraham; Zeeva Adler; Chanie Bandman; Dobi Baum; Krasie Benedikt; Rivky Berger; Surie Berger; Tzivi Bertram; Frida Betesh; Chaya Bodner; Avigayil Brailofsky; Toby Bressler; Ophra Charnas; Miriam Cohen; Yvette Cohen; Paula Cukier; Malka Danziger; Brochie Darabaner; Esther Dayan; Orit Engel; Matty Follman; Debbie Friedman; Leeba Friedman; Yocheved Galy; Estee Greenberg; Toby Greisman; Feiga Gross; Hennie Halpert; Naomi Halpert; Molly Hazan; Bracha Malka Indik; Fayge Indik; Suri Jacobovitch; Miriam Kahan; Rivky Kanarek; Esther Kaplinsky; Surie Kaszirer; Raizy Kaufman; Rivky Kleiman; Leah Kreisworth; Esther Gittel Krishevsky; Zena Krispin; Tzipporah Lapa; Feigi Leibowitz; Ashley Levy; Rivky Ludzker; Rochel Marder; Chumie Meisels; Nechamie Miller; Natalie Minichino; Elise Missry; Yehudis Mueller; Suzy Nadel; Chaya Novoseller; Rachel Novoseller; Naomi Pinter; Blima Prag; Chanie Pruzansky; Tzippy Rabinowitz; Fraidy Rokeach; Gittie Ryback; Rachel Salem; Goldie Schechter; Rivka Leah Schechter; Nisi Schon; Chaykie Schreiber; Frieda Schreiber; Chanie Schwartz; Renee Schwekey; Rivky Senderovic; Laura Shasho; Rosie Shemtov; Hindy Silberberg; Mirel Simcha; Bashi Singer; Sara Bluma Singer; Bayla Stein; Leah Sussman; Leah Trenk; Zeldy Waxman; Hindy Weisberg; Osnas Weitman; Yaffa Yakoel; Idy Yoffe; Cyrille Yurowitz; Raizy Yurowitz.